Complementary and Alternative Medicine in Urology

Guest Editor

MARK A. MOYAD, MD, MPH

UROLOGIC CLINICS OF NORTH AMERICA

www.urologic.theclinics.com

August 2011 • Volume 38 • Number 3

SAUNDERS an imprint of ELSEVIER, Inc.

W.B. SAUNDERS COMPANY
A Division of Elsevier Inc.

1600 John F. Kennedy Blvd. • Suite 1800 • Philadelphia, PA 19103-2899

http://www.theclinics.com

UROLOGIC CLINICS OF NORTH AMERICA Volume 38, Number 3
August 2011 ISSN 0094-0143, ISBN-13: 978-1-4557-1161-1

Editor: Stephanie Donley

Urologic Clinics of North America (ISSN 0094-0143) is published quarterly by Elsevier Inc., 360 Park Avenue South, New York, NY 10010-1710. Months of issue are February, May, August, and November. Business and Editorial Offices: 1600 John F. Kennedy Blvd., Suite 1800, Philadelphia, PA 19103-2899. Periodicals postage paid at New York, NY and additional mailing offices. Subscription prices are $311.00 per year (US individuals), $519.00 per year (US institutions), $363.00 per year (Canadian individuals), $636.00 per year (Canadian institutions), $451.00 per year (foreign individuals), and $636.00 per year (foreign institutions). Foreign air speed delivery is included in all *Clinics* subscription prices. All prices are subject to change without notice. **POSTMASTER:** Send address changes to *Urologic Clinics of North America*, Elsevier Health Sciences Division, Subscription Customer Service, 3251 Riverport Lane, Maryland Heights, MO 63043. Customer Service: 1-800-654-2452 (US). From outside the United States, call 1-314-447-8871. Fax: 1-314-447-8029. E-mail: JournalsCustomerServiceusa@elsevier.com (for print support) and JournalsOnlineSupport-usa@elsevier.com (for online support).

Reprints. For copies of 100 or more, of articles in this publication, please contact the Commercial Reprints Department, Elsevier Inc., 360 Park Avenue South, New York, New York 10010-1710. Tel.: 212-633-3813; Fax: 212-462-1935; E-mail: reprints@elsevier.com.

Urologic Clinics of North America is covered in MEDLINE/PubMed (*Index Medicus*), *Excerpta Medica*, *Current Contents/Clinical Medicine*, *Science Citation Index*, and *ISI/BIOMED*.

Printed and bound by CPI Group (UK) Ltd, Croydon, CR0 4YY

Transferred to Digital Print 2011

Contributors

GUEST EDITOR

MARK A. MOYAD, MD, MPH
Jenkins/Pokempner Director of Preventive and
Alternative Medicine, Department of Urology,
University of Michigan Medical Center, Ann
Arbor, Michigan; Consulting Director of
Medical Education and Research for the
Eisenhower Wellness Institute, Eisenhower
Medical Center, Rancho Mirage, California

AUTHORS

ANDREW L. AVINS, MD, MPH
Clinical Professor, Kaiser Permanente,
Northern California Division of Research,
Oakland, California

CHRISTINE M. BARNETT, MD
Division of Hematology and Medical Oncology,
Knight Cancer Institute, Oregon Health and
Science University, Portland, Oregon

TOMASZ M. BEER, MD
Division of Hematology and Medical Oncology,
Knight Cancer Institute, Oregon Health and
Science University, Portland, Oregon

STEPHEN BENT, MD
Associate Professor, Department of Medicine,
University of California San Francisco,
San Francisco, California

LORIS BORGHI, MD
Full Professor of Internal Medicine and Chief,
Internal Medicine and Subacute Critical Care
Clinic, Department of Clinical Sciences,
University of Parma, Parma, Italy

THOMAS BSCHLEIPFER, MD, PhD
Clinic for Urology, Pediatric Urology and
Andrology, Justus Liebig University Giessen,
Giessen, Germany

JEANNE A. DRISKO, MD
Riordan Endowed Professor of Orthomolecular
Medicine; Director, Program in Integrative
Medicine, University of Kansas Medical
Center, Kansas City, Kansas

REGINALD W. DUSING, MD
Director, Division of Nuclear Medicine;
Associate Professor, Department of Radiology,
Kansas University Medical Center,
Kansas City, Kansas

KATHERINE ESPOSITO, MD, PhD
Associate Professor of Endocrinology and
Metabolism, Department of Cardio-Thoracic
and Respiratory Sciences, Second University
of Naples, Naples, Italy

MICHAEL R. FREEMAN, PhD
The Urological Diseases Research Center;
Enders Research Laboratories, Departments
of Surgery and Biological Chemistry and
Molecular Pharmacology, Children's Hospital
Boston, Harvard Medical School, Boston,
Massachusetts

DARIO GIUGLIANO, MD, PhD
Professor of Endocrinology and Metabolism,
Department of Geriatrics and Metabolic
Diseases, Second University of Naples,
Naples, Italy

GORDON G. GRADO, MD, FACRO, FACR
Medical Director, Southwest Oncology Centers, Scottsdale, Arizona; Wurtele Family Professor in Radiation Oncology, Department of Radiation Oncology, University of Minnesota, Minneapolis, Minnesota

JEFFREY M. HOLZBEIERLEIN, MD
Director, Prostate Cancer Prevention Program; Associate Professor, Department of Urology Surgery, University of Kansas Medical Center, Kansas City, Kansas

CHRISTOPHER J. KANE, MD
Professor of Surgery; Chief of Urology, Division of Urology, Department of Surgery, University of California San Diego, San Diego, California; Urologic Cancer Unit, Moores UCSD Cancer Center, La Jolla, California

LAURENCE H. KLOTZ, MD
Sunnybrook Health Science Centre, Toronto, Ontario, Canada

MARK LEVINE, MD
Chief, Molecular and Clinical Nutrition Section; Senior Staff Physician, National Institutes of Health, Bethesda, Maryland

TIZIANA MESCHI, MD
Aggregate Professor of Internal Medicine, Internal Medicine and Subacute Critical Care Clinic, Department of Clinical Sciences, University of Parma, Parma, Italy

MARK A. MOYAD, MD, MPH
Jenkins/Pokempner Director of Preventive and Alternative Medicine, Department of Urology, University of Michigan Medical Center, Ann Arbor, Michigan; Consulting Director of Medical Education and Research for the Eisenhower Wellness Institute, Eisenhower Medical Center, Rancho Mirage, California

J. CURTIS NICKEL, MD
Professor of Urology; Canada Research Chair in Urologic Pain and Inflammation, Department of Urology, Queen's University, Kingston General Hospital, Kingston, Ontario, Canada

ANTONIO NOUVENNE, MD, PhD
Doctor, Internal Medicine and Subacute Critical Care Clinic, Department of Clinical Sciences, University of Parma, Parma, Italy

ADRIAN PILATZ, MD
Clinic for Urology, Pediatric Urology and Andrology, Justus Liebig University Giessen, Giessen, Germany

OMER A. RAHEEM, MD
Urologic Oncology Research Fellow, Division of Urology, Department of Surgery, University of California San Diego, San Diego, California; Urologic Cancer Unit, Moores UCSD Cancer Center, La Jolla, California

MACK ROACH III, MD
Chair, Radiation Oncology; Professor, Radiation Oncology and Urology, Helen Diller Family Comprehensive Cancer Center, University of California-San Francisco, San Francisco, California

DANIEL A. SHOSKES, MD
Professor of Surgery, Department of Urology, Glickman Urological and Kidney Institute, Cleveland Clinic, Cleveland, Ohio

KEITH R. SOLOMON, PhD
The Urological Diseases Research Center; Enders Research Laboratories, Department of Orthopaedic Surgery, Children's Hospital Boston, Harvard Medical School, Boston, Massachusetts

PETER VAN VELDHUIZEN, MD
Director, Division of Hematology and Oncology; Professor, Department of Internal Medicine, University of Kansas Medical Center, Kansas City, Kansas

FLORIAN M.E. WAGENLEHNER, MD, PhD
Clinic for Urology, Pediatric Urology and Andrology, University Hospital Giessen and Marburg GmbH, Justus Liebig University Giessen, Giessen, Germany

WOLFGANG WEIDNER, MD, PhD
Clinic for Urology, Pediatric Urology and Andrology, Justus Liebig University Giessen, Giessen, Germany

KIRK J. WOJNO, MD
Director of Pathology, Comprehensive Medical Center, Pathology, Royal Oak, Michigan

Contents

Research into the role of cholesterol and prostate disease has been ongoing for many years, but our mechanistic and translational understanding is still poor. Recent evidence indicates that cholesterol-lowering drugs reduce the risk of aggressive prostate cancer. This article reviews the literature on the relationship between circulating cholesterol and prostate cancer. The data strongly point to hypercholesterolemia as a risk factor for prostate cancer progression and suggest clinical opportunities for the use of cholesterol-lowering therapies to alter disease course.

Saw palmetto is widely used to treat lower urinary tract symptoms (LUTS) caused by benign prostatic hyperplasia (BPH). Although there is passionate support for herbal and complementary therapies for LUTS, clinical evidence is mixed. Because there is a well-recognized, profound placebo effect in tests of efficacy for agents treating LUTS, it is imperative that all therapies be tested in placebo-controlled trials. This article reviews evidence of the efficacy and safety of saw palmetto for men with LUTS caused by BPH, with particular emphasis on published randomized clinical trials and the upcoming Complementary and Alternative Medicine for Urologic Symptoms (CAMUS) trial.

Chronic prostatitis/chronic pelvic pain syndrome (CP/CPPS) is a common condition with a heterogeneous origin that responds best to multimodal therapy. The bioflavonoid quercetin has antioxidant and antiinflammatory effects that have proven useful for treating this condition. Using the clinical phenotype system UPOINT, quercetin can be helpful for those with organ-specific complaints (bladder or prostate) and pelvic floor spasm. This article discusses the current understanding of CP/CPPS and how treatment with quercetin can be used alone or as part of multimodal therapy.

Prostatitis syndrome is a frequent condition in men. It is not known in most patients if the prostate is the only organ involved. Therefore, the disease is characterized as chronic prostatitis–chronic pelvic pain syndrome (CP-CPPS). Although many studies have been performed in patients with CP-CPPS, current trial evidence is conflicting and therapeutic options are controversial. Given the need for long-term treatment in CP-CPPS patients, phytotherapeutics, such as pollen extract, are an option due to few side effects. Preclinical studies on pollen extract have shown effects on smooth muscles of the bladder and urethra, strong antiinflammatory effects, and antiproliferative effects.

GOAL STATEMENT
The goal of *Urologic Clinics of North America* is to keep practicing urologists and urology residents up to date with current clinical practice in urology by providing timely articles reviewing the state of the art in patient care.

ACCREDITATION
The *Urologic Clinics of North America* is planned and implemented in accordance with the Essential Areas and Policies of the Accreditation Council for Continuing Medical Education (ACCME) through the joint sponsorship of the University of Virginia School of Medicine and Elsevier. The University of Virginia School of Medicine is accredited by the ACCME to provide continuing medical education for physicians.

The University of Virginia School of Medicine designates this enduring material activity for a maximum of 15 *AMA PRA Category 1 Credit(s)*™ for each issue, 60 credits per year. Physicians should claim only the credit commensurate with the extent of their participation in the activity.

The American Medical Association has determined that physicians not licensed in the US who participate in this CME activity are eligible for a maximum of 15 *AMA PRA Category 1 Credit(s)*™ for each issue, 60 credits per year.

Credit can be earned by reading the text material, taking the CME examination online at http://www.theclinics.com/home/cme, and completing the evaluation. After taking the test, you will be required to review any and all incorrect answers. Following completion of the test and evaluation, your credit will be awarded and you may print your certificate.

FACULTY DISCLOSURE/CONFLICT OF INTEREST
The University of Virginia School of Medicine, as an ACCME accredited provider, endorses and strives to comply with the Accreditation Council for Continuing Medical Education (ACCME) Standards of Commercial Support, Commonwealth of Virginia statutes, University of Virginia policies and procedures, and associated federal and private regulations and guidelines on the need for disclosure and monitoring of proprietary and financial interests that may affect the scientific integrity and balance of content delivered in continuing medical education activities under our auspices.

The University of Virginia School of Medicine requires that all CME activities accredited through this institution be developed independently and be scientifically rigorous, balanced and objective in the presentation/discussion of its content, theories and practices.

All authors/editors participating in an accredited CME activity are expected to disclose to the readers relevant financial relationships with commercial entities occurring within the past 12 months (such as grants or research support, employee, consultant, stock holder, member of speakers bureau, etc.). The University of Virginia School of Medicine will employ appropriate mechanisms to resolve potential conflicts of interest to maintain the standards of fair and balanced education to the reader. Questions about specific strategies can be directed to the Office of Continuing Medical Education, University of Virginia School of Medicine, Charlottesville, Virginia.

The faculty and staff of the University of Virginia Office of Continuing Medical Education have no financial affiliations to disclose.

The authors/editors listed below have identified no professional or financial affiliations for themselves or their spouse/partner:
Andrew L. Avins, MD, MPH; Christine M. Barnett, MD; Stephen Bent, MD; Loris Borghi, MD; Stephanie Donley, (Acquisitions Editor); Jeanne A. Drisko, MD; Reginald W. Dusing, MD; Katherine Esposito, MD, PhD; Michael R. Freeman, PhD; Dario Giugliano, MD, PhD; Laurence H. Klotz, MD; Mark Levine, MD; Tiziana Meschi, MD; Antonio Nouvenne, MD, PhD; Adrian Pilatz, MD; Omer A. Raheem, MD; Keith R. Solomon, PhD; and Peter Van Veldhuizen, MD.

The authors/editors listed below identified the following professional or financial affiliations for themselves or their spouse/partner:
Tomasz M. Beer, MD is a consultant and is a patent holder for Receptor Therapeutics.
Thomas Bschleipfer, MD, PhD is a consultant and is on the Speakers' Bureau for Astellas and Bayer Health Care/Bayer Vital GmbH, and is an industry funded research/investigator for Allergan.
Gordon G. Grado, MD is on the Speakers' Bureau for Brachysciences, and is on the Advisory Board and owns stock for Medytec and Compact Particle Accelerator Corp.
Jeffrey M. Holzbeierlein, MD is on the Speakers Bureau for Endo Pharmaceuticals, Ferring Pharmaceuticals, Centocor Ortho Biotech, and Amgen; is an industry funded research/investigator for Amgen; and is a consultant and is on the Advisory Board for Centocor Ortho Biotech.
Christopher J. Kane, MD is on the Speakers' Bureau for AMGEN and Centocor Ortho Biotech Services LLC, and is a consultant for GENPROBE.
Mark A. Moyad, MD, MPH (Guest Editor) is a consultant for Abbott Labs, Embria Health Sciences, Farr Labs, Guthy Renker, and NBTY; is on the Speakers' Bureau for Abbott Labs; and receives royalties from Guthy Renker.
J. Curtis Nickel, MD is an industry funded research/investigator and a consultant for Glaxo-Smith-Kline, Johnson and Johnson, Pfizer, Watson, Ferring, and Taris Biomedical; and is a consultant for Farr Laboratories, Triton, Cernelle, Cernelle, and Trillium Therapeutics.
Mack Roach III, MD is a Board Member for the American Cancer Society; receives royalties from Up-to-Date, Prostate Cancer; is on the Advisory Board for CareCore, Centocor Ortho Biotech Services, Dendreon, Ferring Pharmaceuticals, Myriad Genetics, and Novartis; receives study support from Molecular Insight; and is on the Spreakers' Bureau for ASTRA-ZENECA and Ferring Pharmaceuticals.
Daniel A. Shoskes, MD is on the Advisory Committee/Board of Farr Labs, and owns stock in Triurol.
William Steers, MD (Test Author) is employed by the American Urologic Association, is a reviewer and consultant for NIH, and is an investigator for Allergan.
Florian M.E. Wagenlehner, MD, PhD is an industry funded research/investigator and a consultant for Strathmann GmbH, Germany and Cernelle, Sweden.
Wolfgang Weidner, MD is an industry funded research/investigator and consultant for Cernelle, Sweden.
Kirk J. Wojno, MD is on the Speakers' Bureau for Aureon Biosciences and Know Error, is a consultant for AmDx Laboratory Sciences, and is an industry funded research/investigator for Dendreon.

Disclosure of Discussion of Non-FDA Approved Uses for Pharmaceutical Products and/or Medical Devices
The University of Virginia School of Medicine, as an ACCME provider, requires that all faculty presenters identify and disclose any off-label uses for pharmaceutical and medical device products. The University of Virginia School of Medicine recommends that each physician fully review all the available data on new products or procedures prior to clinical use.

TO ENROLL
To enroll in the Urologic Clinics of North America Continuing Medical Education program, call customer service at 1-800-654-2452 or visit us online at www.theclinics.com/home/cme. The CME program is available to subscribers for an additional fee of $207.00.

Urologic Clinics of North America

THE CLINICS ARE NOW AVAILABLE ONLINE!

Access your subscription at:
www.theclinics.com

Preface

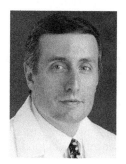

Mark A. Moyad, MD, MPH
Guest Editor

I really cannot believe it has been almost 10 years since I had the pleasure of guest editing a unique issue of *Urologic Clinics of North America* that was one of the first medical journals to ever devote an entire volume of articles to complementary and alternative medicine (CAM) in urology. The issue itself received a lot of attention and was successful, but it was not the easiest task locating multiple authors from around the world to write articles for that edition.

Fast forward to now and everything has changed in regard to CAM and urology. And, when I mean everything, I really mean every single thing. In late 1990s and early 2000s, it was difficult to find individuals working in CAM in any aspect of urology. Of course, there was enormous interest and the occasional lecture at a conference, but now almost every aspect of urology has someone working or conducting research on CAM. Most medical meetings have entire lectures in the area of lifestyle changes and supplements, for example, and almost every conventional treatment lecture that I attend at least references some aspect of healthy lifestyle changes that can be utilized to improve clinical outcomes. Internationally, the landscape has also been positively altered, and this is so wonderful to witness because there are now numerous experts in different areas of urology devoting much of their time to nontraditional treatments that can improve the lives of patients. For example, in this issue, extensive research is summarized on lifestyle changes for kidney stone risk reduction, or male and female sexual dysfunction that will improve clinical practice. Dietary supplement research on nonbacterial prostatitis is also currently a well-covered global

subject. In other words, it has become common today for most major medical centers to vigorously conduct some research in CAM. A decade ago, a medical center was considered different or unique if they were just discussing CAM or offering a community lecture.

Another major evolution in the landscape of medicine and urology is the seemingly exponential increase of over-the-counter (OTC) medicines or options. I am not just talking about supplements but pharmaceutical medicines, which now create a plethora of choices for the consumer that can be quite daunting. Thus, health care professionals, like it or not, have to almost specialize and focus some of their knowledge of what is and is not available for the consumer at the local health food store or pharmacy. The days of being able to just dabble, so to speak, in the area of CAM or OTC medicine are over in my opinion. If you are not dedicating most of your time to this field, it is difficult to be able to provide an adequate overview of the subject. It is no wonder that so many physicians still struggle with this area of medicine in terms of knowledge and expertise. It really has become a full-time job (who would have believed this?).

It has always been interesting to me that in the area of cardiovascular medicine a health care professional can mention that when diet, exercise, and certain supplements are not enough there is always a pharmaceutical solution. However, that is really true of all aspects of preventive medicine right now, so that this should also be the standard in urology. For example, health care professionals can now reference lifestyle and dietary supplement studies in BPH, CPPS (chronic pelvic pain syndrome), ED, FSD, incontinence, stones, urinary

Urol Clin N Am 38 (2011) xi–xii
doi:10.1016/j.ucl.2011.05.005

tract infections, urologic cancers (bladder, kidney, prostate, …), and even to reduce side effects from common treatments such as androgen deprivation therapy. This has to represent one of the greatest changes in urology in recent history. Urology has become the specialty that arguably leads CAM research and knowledge and the SELECT and CAMUS trials are just a hint of this reality. Most pharmaceutical trials in urology are publishing an enormous amount of data on diet and supplements and the PCPT (Prostate Cancer Prevention Trial) is just one example.

Finally, and most importantly, the authors of the articles in this current issue of *Urologic Clinics of North America* represent the future. They are setting standards in this area of medicine that could not have been believed since the last issue. Whether it is imaging, other markers, lifestyle changes, cholesterol, supplements, etc, they are able to find the financing, conduct the novel research, and just devote the needed time to bring respect to this once ignored area of medicine. They and others are also quietly but effectively,

via their actions, teaching others the importance of CAM in urology. It is a remarkable thing to observe, especially when I reach for my 10-year-old previous CAM issue in the *Urologic Clinics of North America* that still sits on my bookshelf at home. Perhaps it is a midlife crisis or just a decade of aging that causes this type of serious reflection on my part. Regardless of the reason, it is an absolute honor and pleasure to continue to watch the transformation of CAM from an occasional area of interest in urology to a full-time discipline that will improve the lives of patients all around the world.

Mark A. Moyad, MD, MPH
Department of Urology
University of Michigan Medical Center
1500 East Medical Center Drive
Ann Arbor, MI 48109-0330, USA

E-mail address:
moyad@umich.edu

The Complex Interplay Between Cholesterol and Prostate Malignancy

Keith R. Solomon, PhD[a,b,]*, Michael R. Freeman, PhD[a,c,d,]*

KEYWORDS

- Prostate cancer • Cholesterol • Statins • Steroidogenesis
- Castration resistance

…it seems that the balance of evidence is…in favor of cholesterol's playing at least some part in the growth of malignant tumors, and… in benign enlargement of the prostate.
—G.I.M. Swyer, 1942

CHOLESTEROL AND PROSTATE CANCER: DECONSTRUCTING A COMPLEX RELATIONSHIP

After more than a hundred years of research into the topic of cholesterol and abnormal cell growth,[1] much debate and substantial doubt remain concerning the effect of hypercholesterolemia on prostate disorders. These unresolved issues include whether drugs used to treat hypercholesterolemia alter the risk of prostate cancer. Much of the controversy stems from limitations in the existing literature and interpretations thereof that go beyond the data. This review highlights some of these points of debate and draws contrasts between established findings, inconsistencies between randomized trials and observational studies, and what we believe to be misinterpretations of published data sets. What emerges from a careful analysis of a large body of literature, going back many decades, is an integration of older findings and data in newer reports that supports a conclusion that hypercholesterolemia is a risk factor for aggressive prostate cancer.

The prostate synthesizes cholesterol at rates equivalent to the liver and an age-dependent shift in cholesterol homeostasis allows cholesterol to accumulate in the prostate at high levels in older individuals.[2] Cholesterol makes up about 30% of the lipid content of plasma membranes and is an absolute requirement for new membrane synthesis. This neutral lipid also contributes to the physiologic properties of cell membranes by regulating membrane fluidity, promoting negative membrane curvature, and by interdigitating with acyl chains of phospholipids to create liquid ordered membrane microdomains. Cholesterol-rich microdomains are believed to play an important role in signal transduction and in other physiologic

Conflict of interest: The authors have nothing to disclose.
This study was supported by grants from the NIH (R01CA101046 to K.R.S.; R01CA143777 to M.R.F.) and the US Department of Defense (W81XWH-08-1-0150 to M.R.F.).
[a] The Urological Diseases Research Center, Boston, MA, USA
[b] Enders Research Laboratories, Department of Orthopaedic Surgery, Children's Hospital Boston, Harvard Medical School, 300 Longwood Avenue, Boston, MA 02115, USA
[c] Enders Research Laboratories, Department of Surgery, Children's Hospital Boston, Harvard Medical School, 300 Longwood Avenue, Boston, MA 02115, USA
[d] Department of Biological Chemistry and Molecular Pharmacology, Harvard Medical School, 300 Longwood Avenue, Boston, MA 02115, USA
* Corresponding authors. Enders Research Laboratories, The Urological Diseases Research Center, Children's Hospital Boston, Harvard Medical School, 300 Longwood Avenue, Boston, MA 02115.
E-mail addresses: keith.solomon@childrens.harvard.edu; michael.freeman@childrens.harvard.edu

Urol Clin N Am 38 (2011) 243–259
doi:10.1016/j.ucl.2011.04.001

mechanisms such as solute transport. Because of the multiple roles of cholesterol in the cell, perturbations in cholesterol metabolism might conceivably alter epithelial, stromal, and inflammatory cell infiltrates in the prostate. In a scenario involving rapid cell proliferation, the requirement for cholesterol assembly into new membranes may be a rate-limiting step in the process of tissue growth. Tumor cell proliferation, in turn, may affect circulating cholesterol levels. This article reviews various aspects of this complex relationship.

CANCER AND ITS EFFECTS ON CIRCULATING CHOLESTEROL: THE U-SHAPED CURVE

The concept of the U-shaped curve refers to the higher levels of mortality found on either end of the cholesterol level spectrum that many investigators discovered when studies were performed to assess the potential relationship between circulating cholesterol and mortality. Although it is well established that the increase in mortality at the high end of the cholesterol spectrum is caused by cardiovascular disease, the higher level of mortality at the low end of the spectrum is more mysterious and seems to emanate from a variety of sources. These sources include an unexplained higher frequency of accidental deaths in individuals with low cholesterol and an association between endemic hepatitis and low cholesterol. However, another important reason for higher mortality at the low end of the U arises from the cholesterol-lowering effect of cancer itself; therefore, the low end of the curve likely includes an excess of individuals with preexisting cancer.

Although earlier articles speculated on this point, evidence implicating a direct effect of cholesterol lowering on increased cancer risk was first reported in 1971 by Pearce and Dayton.[3] These investigators examined cancer incidence and cancer-specific deaths in 2 patient cohorts, one that received a control diet and the other an experimental cholesterol-lowering diet. The experimental diet was essentially the same as control, but with less cholesterol and with additional polyunsaturated fats. These investigators found that within 10 years of initiation of the study there was more total cancer (81 vs 66), more cancer deaths (31 vs 17), and, for our purposes, more prostate cancers (12 vs 10) in the experimental diet cohort, although the prostate cancer differences are small. A review of 5 diet trials published in 1971[4] did not support a cholesterol-lowering diet and cancer association (odds ratio [OR] for cancer incidence was 1.15 95% confidence interval [CI] [0.81–1.63]; for cancer death it was 1.08 95% CI [0.71–1.69]) and other, subsequent, cholesterol-lowering diet trials did not confirm the observations of Pearce and Dayton.[5] A review of prestatin cholesterol-lowering trials in 1988,[6] in which 22 randomized trials including ≈40,000 individuals were discussed (only 2 of which are cited), found no evidence suggesting an association between low cholesterol and cancer risk. This finding contrasts with a 1990 meta-analysis[7] of 6 cholesterol-lowering trials, which used stringent criteria for selection of included studies. This review reported a significant increase in overall cancer mortality (OR 1.43 95% CI [1.08–1.90]) that remained even when studies not including drugs (2 studies) were used in the analysis (OR 1.62 95% [CI 1.03–2.57]).

Randomized, placebo-controlled or diet-controlled cholesterol-lowering trials were largely equivocal in their conclusions concerning a cholesterol-cancer association, and population studies were equally ambiguous. Rose and colleagues[8] pooled data from 6 prospective population studies (more on these studies later) to show a low cholesterol-colon cancer link, with patients with cancer of the colon having on average a 10-mg/dL reduction in total cholesterol versus the population mean. The conclusions of this early study were buttressed by several additional population studies that showed excess cancers in the cohorts with the lowest cholesterol.

We have reviewed 52 population studies[9–60] that reported on cholesterol and total cancer incidence and/or mortality that were published from 1972 to 2009. In total, these reports cover 79.5 million men and women ages 15 to 99 years (average 38–63 years) from Finland, Yugoslavia, the United States, New Zealand, Italy, France, Japan, China, Scotland, England, Norway, Israel, Australia, and Sweden. Thirty-two studies report an inverse association between cancer risk and cholesterol level, 16 show no association, 2 provided no statistics, 1 was a follow-up report, and 1 study was largely equivocal. Studies that report excess risk usually find this association more prominently in men and, most frequently, the associated cancers are those of the liver, colon, and lung (probably because of the high rates of mortality seen with these cancers). Many of these studies were long in duration (as long as 40 years); consequently, some of the investigators transformed the data by removing cancer cases that appeared in the early years of the studies (defined by investigators as those occurring anywhere from 2 to 20 years after study initiation). In 12 of a total of 30 of these reports, removal of cancers that appeared early in the study either diminished or eliminated the significance of the low cholesterol-increased cancer risk association, suggesting that lower cholesterol was not the cause but the result of cancer.

One intriguing aspect of these population studies that seems to strongly support the hypothesis that the inverse correlation between cancer and cholesterol level is caused by an effect of cancer on cholesterol level is that there is no absolute low level of cholesterol associated with cancer. For example, an association is found when the low cholesterol level for a population is $\leq 230^{26}$ or $\leq 134^{25}$ (ie, the 20% of any cohort with the lowest cholesterol in any population seems to have a greater prevalence of cancer than groups within that population with higher cholesterol). Logically, one would predict that if low cholesterol triggered cancer it would do so at a relatively uniform cholesterol level, and that if such an association existed, populations with low cholesterol would show an excess of certain cancers, an outcome that population studies do not support. Instead, if cancer reduces cholesterol level we would expect the 20% of the population with the lowest cholesterol to have excess cancer regardless of the endemic cholesterol level of the population, a prediction that is supported by the population studies when considered in aggregate.

A second point that seems to show that low cholesterol is the result of the effect of cancer on the host, and not the cause of cancer, arises from studies that measured cholesterol proximal to time of death. Keys and colleagues[25] show that men who died of cancer within 2 years of study onset had cholesterol values 9.48% lower than the average of all men at entry. Sherwin and colleagues[44] reported that men who developed cancer exhibited a 22.7-mg/dL drop in cholesterol level versus matched survivors. The International Collaborative Group showed that individuals dying from cancer 1 year after cholesterol measurement had cholesterol levels that were 24 to 35 mg/dL lower than controls (ie, those not dying); those dying 2 to 5 years after cholesterol measure reported values that were 4 to 5 mg/dL lower than controls; and those dying of cancer 6 to 10 years after cholesterol measure had cholesterol values 2 mg/dL lower than controls.[10] These findings likely reflect the tendency of cancer to depress circulating cholesterol levels.

Particularly revealing are studies of cholesterol level variation over time in relation to cancer incidence or death. There are only a few of these reports because they require multiple cholesterol measures over time and few studies were designed to capture these data. The first such report we analyzed is by Sorlei and Feinleib,[46] which used Framingham Heart Study data and showed that in some individuals who develop cancer, cholesterol levels are lower than the mean value up to 18 years before cancer diagnosis, whereas in other individuals cholesterol levels decline near the time of diagnosis. The robustness of the analysis is hampered because the investigators split the group by decades of age and sex, thus making each cohort small. The investigators write "Although the Framingham data are not conclusive, they do suggest that in some cancer cases where the serum cholesterol level was lower than that expected at as much as 16–18 years before cancer diagnosis, the depressed level was likely to be a precursor to the tumor growth. However, consistent with the metabolic consequences of tumor growth, the data show that in some cancer cases, serum cholesterol had decreased at measurements made close to the time of cancer diagnosis." Pekkanen and colleagues,[33] studying Finnish men (aged 55–74 years) analyzed the change in cholesterol levels from 1959 to 1974 (every 5 years) in individuals who did not have cardiovascular disease in 1974. The investigators found that older men (aged 65–74 years in 1974) with the steepest decline in cholesterol had a higher risk of dying from cancer. In 1992 Pocock and Seed[37] reported cholesterol time trend data from British men and women with hypertension (aged 65–74 years) reporting that cholesterol levels fell an average of 11.2 mg/dL in men within a year before a cancer death. Sharp and Pocock,[42] again using Framingham Heart Study data, report several highly relevant findings: (1) 61% of individuals have a 12.6 mg/dL (95% CI [8.46–16.70]) decline in cholesterol within 2 years before a cancer death; (2) the mean level of cholesterol 2 to 4 years before death from cancer is 10 mg/dL lower than the population norm; (3) the odds of dying of cancer within 4 years were increased (2.11 95% CI [1.41–3.14]) in individuals whose decline in cholesterol was greater than 38 mg/dL.

Whether low cholesterol causes cancer or low cholesterol is the result of cancer has important implications for public health. Not surprisingly, the National Institutes of Health (NIH) was concerned, especially in light of the large body of evidence that high cholesterol is associated with death from cardiovascular disease (nearly all the population studies of cholesterol and mortality verified this) and the international reaction to reduce cholesterol levels broadly in the human population. At least 3 NIH conferences[61,62] were held to explore the relationship between cholesterol and mortality, and cancer mortality specifically: the first was held in February of 1980, and the second soon after in May of the same year[61]; a third was held in October of 1990.[62] Because the report of Jacobs and colleagues[62] is the most thorough, with its inclusion of 19 population studies in its analysis, we briefly explore this report with regards to cancer. After elimination of cancer deaths occurring within 5 years of the onset of each individual study, the cancer rate ratio for men with cholesterol less than 160 mg/dL was between 1.18 ($P<.05$) and 1.23 ($P<.001$), depending on how the studies were analyzed. For women the cancer rate ratio was 1.05 (not significant). Significant associations between low cholesterol and cancer were found for lung cancer in both men and women, and other cancers (not specified) in women. No association was found between low cholesterol and colon cancer. The summarized conclusion from the 3 NIH-sponsored conferences was that there were insufficient data regarding the association between cholesterol and cancer. They cite multiple concerns, including (1) the modest increase in cancer among the low-cholesterol population, (2) the lack of a clear association in women, (3) the presence of the cancer-cholesterol association in some populations but not in others, (4) the presence of a presumptive effect in some but not all studies, and (5) the absence of a plausible biologic mechanism that would explain why lower, but still physiologic, levels of cholesterol might trigger cancer. These considerations, as well as an absence of information about the effect of disease on cholesterol levels over time, prevented the conferees at any of the 3 meetings mentioned earlier from adopting specific recommendations on cholesterol reduction therapy. The recommendation of all 3 NIH conferences on low cholesterol and mortality was not to alter the prescription of lowering cholesterol levels to improve public health, but to continue to study the issue.

The concern that low cholesterol might increase cancer risk persisted until the early 1990s; however, it has almost entirely disappeared in the poststatin era. Multiple meta-analyses report that statins, which potently reduce cholesterol levels, do not cause an increase in cancer.[63–65] This finding leaves the conclusion that cancer itself reduces circulating cholesterol as the only plausible explanation for the presumptive associations reported in the population studies described earlier.

What do the large population studies of overall disease incidence, mortality, and cholesterol level, in which prostate cancer was not an exclusive focus, indicate about prostate cancer, specifically? A small minority of the studies (10 of 52 publications) we examined for this review include prostate cancer in the analysis, and the total number of prostate cancer cases combined in the studies is only 1652. The following discussion summarizes all of the major population studies that include prostate cancer as an end point. Knect and colleagues[26] reported a positive association between low cholesterol and increased prostate cancer risk (n = 45),

but did not follow their cohort for greater than 5 years. Kark and colleagues[24] found that individuals with prostate cancer (n = 12) had significantly reduced cholesterol levels. Hiatt and Fireman[19] reported on 601 prostate cancers and found that removing cases occurring within the first 2 years after study inception eliminated the positive correlation between low cholesterol and cancer incidence. Williams and colleagues[53] reported on 44 prostate cancer cases, but do not comment specifically on a cholesterol-prostate cancer association. Wingard and colleagues[54] reported on 49 prostate cancer cases, but found no cholesterol-cancer association. Morris and colleagues[31] found a significant low-cholesterol–cancer association (n = 26). These investigators show that the 5-year prostate cancer incidence rates decreased stepwise with lower to higher cholesterol levels (6.9 deaths/1000 cases when cholesterol was ≤204 mg/dL; 6.5/1000 in the 205–230 mg/dL quartile; 2.2/1000 in the 231–260 mg/dL quartile and 1.7 deaths/1000 cases in the ≥261 mg/dL quartile). Schatzkin and colleagues[40] reported on 95 prostate cancer deaths and found no cholesterol-cancer association. Tulinius and colleagues[49] describe no statistically significant association between cholesterol level and 524 incident prostate cancer cases. Davey-Smith and colleagues[45] reported on 92 prostate cancer deaths and in quintile analysis report a nonsignificant trend, with lower levels of cholesterol associated with reduced cancer risk; the hazard ratio (HR) corresponding to a 1 standard deviation decline in cholesterol was 0.85 (95% CI 0.69–1.04). Iso and colleagues found no low cholesterol-prostate cancer association in their 164 cases; instead they report a significant trend of higher levels of cholesterol associated with increased cancer risk (p for trend 0.0023), an association that disappeared when advanced cancers were removed from the analysis (p for trend 0.12). Collectively, these studies point to a modest association between low cholesterol and increased prostate cancer risk.

In contrast to the reports cited earlier that include limited numbers of prostate cancer cases, for the most part were of short duration, and almost never report or comment on late-stage disease (except as it pertains to death), studies that specifically address the potential association between serum cholesterol level and prostate cancer have large enough cohort sizes to allow a more thorough analysis. Thompson and colleagues[66] found no cholesterol-prostate cancer association (n = 100). The Asia Pacific Cohort Studies Collaboration[67] reported on 308 prostate cancer deaths and found a greater number of deaths in the population with the highest cholesterol based on tertile analysis, but the difference was not significant (possibly because of small numbers). Platz and colleagues[68] in a case-control analysis of men in the Health Professionals Follow-up Study reported that men (n = 698) with low cholesterol (Q1 in quartile analysis; cholesterol level is undefined because of assay complications) had a lower risk of high-grade prostate cancer (OR, 0.61 95% CI [0.39–0.98]). Platz and colleagues[69] examined 1251 incident prostate cancers and found that men with low cholesterol (<200 mg/dL) had a lower risk of high-grade disease (Gleason 8–10; OR, 0.41 95% CI [0.22–0.77]). Mondul and colleagues[70] examined 438 incident prostate cancers and determined that men with cholesterol lower than 240 mg/dL were less likely to develop high-grade prostate cancer then men with cholesterol greater than 240 mg/dL, results that were unchanged after eliminating cholesterol-lowering drug users. Batty and colleagues,[71] in a study that included 578 prostate cancer deaths, reported a greater number of cancer-specific deaths in the highest cholesterol tertile (<175 mg/dL HR 1.0 [reference population]; 175–214 mg/dL HR 1.07 95% CI [0.87–1.32]; >214 mg/dL HR 1.35 95% CI [1.11–1.65] p-value for trend = 0.003). These reports do not support a low cholesterol-increased prostate cancer risk association, but instead suggest that men with high cholesterol are either at increased risk for prostate cancer or castrate-resistant disease.

A QUESTION OF PROSTATE-SPECIFIC ANTIGEN

The answer to the question of why some studies support an association between low cholesterol and prostate cancer, whereas others support an association with high cholesterol, most likely reflects when the study was conducted. The US Food and Drug Administration approved serum prostate-specific antigen (PSA) as a prostate cancer biomarker in 1994, forever changing the diagnostic landscape in the field. With PSA testing, men now generally present clinically with early stage disease, years before any clinical symptoms would otherwise appear. Thus, cancer populations considered in studies published before 1994 include many more advanced cancers than studies published in the last 10 years. This important milestone also suggests that cholesterol readings in the pre-PSA era have a greater chance of being a product of tumor metabolism, leading to a low cholesterol-cancer association, whereas cholesterol measures in post-PSA studies are more likely to reflect the cholesterol environment before the development of cancer. This finding would lead to a positive correlation between high cholesterol and prostate cancer risk.

We propose a unifying model that reconciles the data from the pre-PSA and post-PSA studies (**Fig. 1**). The most recent evidence indicates that high circulating cholesterol is a risk factor for prostate cancer.[72] In the pre-PSA era a low cholesterol reading is more likely to be associated with a higher risk of a prostate cancer death; in the post-PSA era this association is reversed. This contradiction can be explained by the different patient cohorts (with regard to extent of disease progression) analyzed in the older versus the new studies, by preclinical findings that high circulating cholesterol promotes prostate growth[73,74] cancer, and by epidemiologic data showing higher cholesterol levels increase prostate cancer risk. Additional evidence includes the apparent protective effects of long-term statin drug therapy on prostate cancer risk (considered later).

However, there are important caveats that alter this simple equation, and these are best understood by considering the period of time between a low cholesterol measure and a prostate cancer diagnosis versus the relative risk of prostate cancer death (see **Fig. 1**). In both the pre-PSA and post-PSA eras a low cholesterol measure within 1 year of a prostate cancer diagnosis raises the risk of a prostate cancer death, whereas in both the pre-PSA and post-PSA eras a low cholesterol measure more than 6 years before a prostate cancer diagnosis reduces the risk of a prostate cancer death (see **Fig. 1**, left end of the curves vs the right end of the curves). Between 1 and approximately 6 years before a prostate cancer diagnosis the tendency for low cholesterol to correlate with increased risk of prostate cancer death is different in the pre-PSA and post-PSA eras. In the pre-PSA era a low cholesterol measure about 1 to 6 years

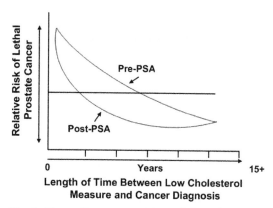

Fig. 1. Theoretic representation of the relationship between low cholesterol and the risk of prostate cancer death in the pre-PSA and post-PSA eras.

before prostate cancer diagnosis raises the risk of a prostate cancer death, whereas in the post-PSA era a low cholesterol measure ~1 to 6 years before a prostate cancer diagnosis decreases the risk of prostate cancer death.

THE STATIN CONTROVERSY

Recent epidemiologic studies from several groups have shown that cholesterol-lowering drugs (primarily 3-hydroxy-3-methylglutaryl coenzyme A [HMG CoA] reductase inhibitors, known as statins) may lower prostate cancer risk, and in particular, the risk of advanced disease.[75–87] Platz and colleagues[84] assessed potential statin drug effects specifically on prostate cancer in an analysis powered to measure differences in cancer incidence and progression in 2579 cancer cases, with 316 cases of advanced disease. The adjusted relative risk of castration-resistant cancer among statin users in this study was 0.51 95% CI (0.30–0.86) and of metastatic or fatal disease was 0.39 95% CI (0.19–0.77) for statin users versus nonusers. These investigators also showed that risk of advanced disease was lower with longer statin use (the relative risk for statin users of <5 years of use was 0.60 95% CI [0.35–1.03] and for ≥5 years of use was 0.26 95% CI [0.08–0.83]). In contrast to advanced disease, this study found no association between statin use and prostate cancer risk, suggesting that incidence alone is inadequate for evaluating potential chemopreventives in this disease.

Several more recent prospective studies from independent groups have largely confirmed the conclusions of Platz and colleagues[79,82–84] that statins reduce the risk of aggressive prostate cancer. Flick and colleagues performed a case-control analysis using a population of 69,047 participants in the California Men's Health Study that included 888 total cases of prostate cancer, with 131 advanced cases. They concluded that use of statins for ≥5 years was associated with a 28% lower disease risk (adjusted rate ratio of 0.72 95% CI [0.53–0.99]). Jacobs and colleagues reported on a case-control study using 55,454 men from the Cancer Prevention Study II Nutrition Cohort, which included 3413 cases of prostate cancer, with 317 cases of advanced disease. This group did not show a change in overall prostate cancer risk in the statin group; however, they found a marginally significant effect on advanced disease among the statin users (adjusted rate ratio of 0.60 95% CI [0.36–1.00]). Murtola and colleagues presented a case-control study of a large study population using data from the Finnish Cancer Registry, the Population Register Center, and the Social

Insurance Institution of Finland (24,723 cases with an equal number of matched controls). This group found a significant reduction of risk of advanced prostate cancer in users of atorvastatin, lovastatin, and simvastatin (approximately 77% of the statin drug usage in the cohort), with an adjusted OR of 0.61 95% CI (0.37–0.98); 0.61 95% CI (0.430.85); and 0.78 95% CI (0.61–1.01), respectively (the overall OR for all statins was 0.75 95% CI [0.62–0.91]). Murtola and colleagues also noted that nonstatin cholesterol-reducing drugs (fibrates specifically) modestly reduced the risk of advanced prostate cancer, but these data did not reach significance, possibly a result of a small sample size. We have proposed that the chemopreventive effects of statin drugs arise predominantly or exclusively from cholesterol lowering, not from other statin effects, such as inhibition of isoprenoid synthesis[72]; consequently, if this hypothesis is true, we would expect that other methods of cholesterol reduction would also modify risk. Recent observational studies of statin effects on prostate cancer risk, which contain large numbers of subjects, are largely supportive of the hypothesis that statins reduce the risk of advanced prostate cancer.

Although the recent literature indicates that long-term statin therapy is chemopreventive against aggressive prostate cancer, large randomized trials of statin drugs that report on cancer (including prostate cancer) do not support this claim.[63–65] There are several reasons that these 2 types of studies tend to present different pictures regarding prostate cancer risk and statin use.

Large randomized, placebo-controlled trials of statins include small numbers of prostate cancers. We reviewed 49[88–136] trial reports that included 134,516 individuals and identified only 5 prostate cancer deaths and 1142 incident prostate cancer cases, and these trials were of short duration (4.2 years on average). Observational studies of prostate cancer risk and statin use include many more prostate cancer cases (77,325 in a total study population of 4,168,049), and they include follow-up to 14 years. This situation explains some of the discrepancy between randomized, placebo-controlled studies and observational studies, but there are some additional important differences that deserve attention.

TOO MUCH PRAVASTATIN?

Of the 34 separate randomized, placebo-controlled trials that we analyzed that reported on the low-density lipoprotein (LDL) reduction, including all the major statin trials (some of the 49 reports we evaluated were various analyses of the same initial trial, and others did not report on LDL reduction), 14 were trials of pravastatin,[90–93,101,102,105,110–112,114,116,119,121,123,127,128,135,136] 6 were simvastatin trials,[88,89,94,96,98,100,118,129,130,133,134] 6 were atorvastatin trials,[99,113,115,117,120,126,131] 4 were trials of fluvastatin,[107–109,124,125] 3 were lovastatin trials,[97,103,106,132] and 1 was a rosuvastatin trial (**Table 1**).[104] Of the 56,095 individuals randomized to any statin, 46.5% were randomized to pravastatin. This situation contrasts greatly with statins used as reported in the observational studies, in which only 1.6% of the patients took pravastatin. This lower percentage of pravastatin is more similar to overall statin sales in which pravastatin represents only about 6% of the total.[72] It is important to note this large difference in the use of a specific statin between these 2 types of reports. Statins are usually considered as an undifferentiated group in population studies, as if 1 statin drug was chemically and physiologically equivalent to another. However, statins are chemically diverse and have significantly different potencies with respect to cholesterol lowering. This large difference in pravastatin use in the various studies may have important consequences with regards to outcomes.

Pravastatin is the weakest of the statin drugs in terms of its ability to inhibit HMG CoA reductase (IC_{50} [half maximal inhibitory concentration] 6.93 nM; Ki 23×10^{-10})[72] and consequently does not reduce total or LDL cholesterol to the same extent as other statins. This difference in potency seems to be reflected in the results of randomized studies of statin effects on cardiovascular disease. Although all statins seem to be similarly effective in reducing risk of cardiovascular disease, pravastatin was less effective than any other statin used in reducing LDL cholesterol (see **Table 1**). In our analysis of these published data, pravastatin reduced LDL by an average of 24.3%. In contrast, simvastatin reduced LDL cholesterol by 32.5%, a difference that is statistically significant ($P = .01$). Moreover, we calculated that the total percentage decline in LDL from all the randomized studies was 28.5%. However, if the patients randomized to take a statin were given statins in the percentage used in observational studies, we estimate that the decrease in LDL cholesterol would be about 32%, a potential difference of 3.5 mg/dL in LDL levels. Because so many patients were randomized to pravastatin, pharmacologic cholesterol lowering in the study population is not so great as would be expected if the patients were taking statins outside the study setting (ie, in the proportions used by the general public). The consequences of this skewed mix of statins for detecting a statin effect on cancer incidence or progression is unknown. However, coupled with the short duration of most randomized studies, patient crossover from placebo to statin (as required by usual care), and patient selection bias (as we discussed in previous works),[72,137] this finding could explain the differences in statin association with prostate cancer risk in randomized, placebo-controlled studies and observational studies.

HOW DOES CHOLESTEROL INCREASE THE RISK OF LETHAL PROSTATE CANCER?

As mentioned earlier, cholesterol plays a vital role in establishing the properties of functional animal cell membranes. It also affects various signaling pathways and proteins, either by direct conjugation to proteins (ie, sonic hedgehog), or by modifying the

Table 1
Number of randomized, placebo-controlled statin trials that recorded LDL reduction, and percentage of LDL reduction achieved. LDL reduction was calculated by subtracting the levels after treatment with pretreatment values in the statin cohort.[1,13,88–93,95–97,99–102,104,106,107,109,110,113–117,119–122,124–128,130–132,135,136] In some studies, the placebo group also showed LDL reduction. In these cases this value was subtracted from the reduction achieved in the treatment group

Statin Trials	Number of Studies	LDL Reduction (%)
Pravastatin	14	24.3 ± 6.5
Simvastatin	6	32.6 ± 8.8
Atorvastatin	6	33.4 ± 8.9
Fluvastatin	4	25.5 ± 9.3
Lovastatin	3	30.6 ± 8.6
Rosuvastatin	1	41

activities of membrane proximal signaling pathways and proteins such as the cell survival kinase, AKT.[138,139] Certain signal transduction pathways seem to be highly sensitive to manipulations in circulating cholesterol levels.[73,74] In vivo, hypercholesterolemia causes increased tumor angiogenesis, reduces tumor apoptosis, and increases tumor cell proliferation.[73,74] The relative contribution(s) of these mechanisms to prostate cancer progression is unknown. We have extensively reviewed these mechanisms in previous commentaries.[72,140–143]

Recent studies have provided another mechanism for tumor-promoting effects of cholesterol that is highly relevant to prostate cancer. Prostate tumors respond to circulating androgen through the action of the androgen receptor (AR), a nuclear receptor that drives prostate cancer cell proliferation and survival even under conditions of hormone suppression during late-stage disease.[144–146] Androgen deprivation therapy[144,147] (ADT) remains the primary treatment strategy for advanced prostate cancer. Despite widespread early responses to therapy, prostate cancer almost invariably becomes castration resistant and the tumor cells continue to grow despite circulating androgen at castrate levels.[144,145] In this phase of disease (termed castration-resistant prostate cancer [CRPC]), tumors become more aggressive. There are several theories about how this castration-resistant phenotype comes about: (1) gene amplification and/or mutation of the AR, allowing the receptor to be sensitive to low levels of androgen[148–154]; (2) residual androgen production from the adrenal glands[155]; and (3) promiscuous receptor-ligand interactions.[150,156]

Although it was 30 years ago that Geller and colleagues[157] first reported that sufficient androgen to drive the AR remained in the prostate after ADT,[157,158] the significance of this observation was partially obscured because other work appeared to show that coadministration of the antiandrogen flutamide, along with castration, totally ablated dihydrotestosterone (DHT) activity, suggesting that any residual disease is not driven by androgen, per se. This latter finding was based on an n = 4 and used an assay that did not detect DHT levels less than 300 pg/g tissue.[159] The combination of castration with an antiandrogen is commonly used to treat advanced prostate cancer. Results of a phase III trial using the CYP17 inhibitor, abiraterone, in men with CRPC showed a significant overall survival benefit, strongly suggesting that for many men, CRPC is still driven, at least in part, by androgen.[160–167] Several groups have presented data showing that prostate tumors in men receiving ADT contain androgen levels high enough to activate the AR.[157,159–166,168–175]

CHOLESTEROL AND ANDROGEN SYNTHESIS

One major biologic role of cholesterol is as the precursor for the synthesis of steroid hormones, including androgens. Enzymes and other proteins are essential in converting cholesterol into testosterone and DHT including steroidogenic acute regulatory protein, obligatory for cholesterol transport into the mitochondria, CYP11A1 to convert cholesterol to pregnenolone, CYP17A and HSD3B to form androstenedione, and a 17β-hydroxysteroid dehydrogenase (eg, AKR1C3 or HSD17B3) to convert androstenedione to testosterone.

Several lines of evidence indicate that prostate cancer cells in vivo synthesize their own androgens (ie, de novo steroidogenesis), including in the castrate environment,[173,176,177] in sufficient quantities to be biologically active. Locke and colleagues[176] reported that all of the enzymes necessary for de novo androgen synthesis are expressed in LNCaP tumor xenografts, and that androgen-starved prostate cancer cells are capable of synthesizing DHT from acetic acid, suggesting that the entire pathway from acetate → cholesterol → DHT is intact in this model system.[176] Montgomery and colleagues[173] reported that the full complement of enzymes comprising the steroidogenic pathways is present in most human primary and metastatic prostate cancers examined, implying that de novo androgen synthesis is not merely an experimental phenomenon, but rather a potential underlying cause of disease progression in the CRPC phase of the disease.

The ability of prostate cancer cells to synthesize androgen from cholesterol may increase after hormone suppression because castration increases serum cholesterol levels,[172,178–181] and because cholesterol synthesis increases in experimental prostatic tumors in the castrate condition.[182] We have noted this increase in serum cholesterol in castrated mice. We have found that hypercholesterolemia accelerates the growth of human prostate cancer xenografts after castration (**Fig. 2**). New data from our group (Mostaghel and colleagues, manuscript in preparation) suggest that hypercholesterolemia contributes to androgen synthesis in prostate tumors, even in the castrate environment. Thus, the combination of castration and an increase in circulating cholesterol may increase the risk of CRPC progression.

In humans, there are 2 potential sources of intratumoral androgens in the castrate environment; they are either products of the adrenal glands (potentially as both precursors and as androgens), or they are created de novo through intratumoral steroidogenesis. After day 14.5 of embryogenesis,[183] adrenal glands in the mouse begin to

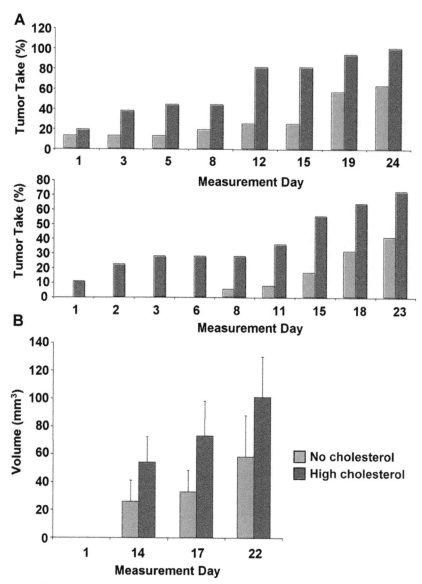

Fig. 2. Tumor growth in castrated mice. Castrated mice were fed isocaloric no-cholesterol or high-cholesterol diets for 80 days. LNCaP cells were subsequently injected subcutaneously and the animals continued on their respective diets for 22 days. (*A*) Tumor take. The numbers of tumor in each diet group were counted and the data are plotted as tumor take (% of all implantation sites) versus time (days). Significance was determined by logistic regression analysis. At all time points at which tumors were present, the 2 cohorts differed significantly ($P<.05$) (n = 40/group). (*B*) Longitudinal volume measurements. Tumors were measured at various time points by calipers starting at first appearance (day 1) and continued until tumor burden required the animals to be killed (day 22). Data are plotted as tumor volume (mm^3) per site versus time (days) ± standard error (n = 40/group).

lose expression of 17α-hydroxylase (CYP17) and express little to none of the enzyme into adulthood. CYP17 is an essential enzyme required to convert pregnenolone to androstenedione, and consequently the murine adrenals produce little to no androgen or androgen precursors (eg, androstenediol).[176,184] The lack of CYP17 in the adrenals of mice also explains why the major glucocorticoid present in the mouse is corticosterone instead of cortisol.[185] In total, these data suggest, provocatively, that in the murine castrate environment prostatic tumors acquire the ability to synthesize T and DHT from intratumoral cholesterol, and do not require adrenal contributions. Whether this is also true in human patients remains to be established.

Cholesterol plays an essential role in steroidogenesis through its place as the precursor for all steroid hormones. However, we propose that cholesterol also plays an additional role as a steroidogenesis pathway agonist. Free cholesterol is cytotoxic and cells have multiple methods of reducing excess free cholesterol including: (1) upregulating the cholesterol efflux transporters, ABCA1, ABCG1, and ABCA7; (2) upregulating enzymes catalyzing the nonhepatic acid pathway of bile acid synthesis, CYP27A1 and CYP7B1[186]; (3) reducing expression of cholesterol receptors LDLR and SR-B1; (4) increasing cholesterol esterification through acyl-CoA cholesterol acyl transferase; and (5) reducing cholesterol synthesis through regulation of HMG CoA reductase expression. In addition, we propose that an additional mechanism for reducing the pool of free cholesterol is through the upregulation of the proteins/enzymes responsible for synthesizing androgens from cholesterol (ie, de novo steroidogenesis within the tumor microenvironment). The relevance of these diverse mechanisms to prostate cancer remains to be tested in experimental models and in humans.

SUMMARY

Circulating cholesterol is a likely risk factor for aggressive prostate cancer. The multifaceted nature of the complex metabolic pathways in which cholesterol participates allows this lipid to play multiple roles in cancer progression. Further studies on the detailed mechanisms of cholesterol effects on prostate and other cancers are warranted, and could lead to new avenues for therapeutic intervention, particularly in controlling progression to late-stage disease.

REFERENCES

1. White RM. On the occurrence of crystals in tumours. J Pathol Bacteriol 1909;13:310.
2. Schaffner CP. Prostatic cholesterol metabolism: regulation and alteration. Prog Clin Biol Res Am 1981;75:279–324.
3. Pearce ML, Dayton S. Incidence of cancer in men on a diet high in polyunsaturated fat. Lancet 1971;1(7697):464–7.
4. Ederer F, Leren P, Turpeinen O, et al. Cancer among men on cholesterol-lowering diets: experience from five clinical trials. Lancet 1971;2(7717): 203–6.
5. Miettinen M, Turpeinen O, Karvonen MJ, et al. Effect of cholesterol-lowering diet on mortality from coronary heart-disease and other causes. A twelve-year clinical trial in men and women. Lancet 1972;2(7782):835–8.
6. Yusuf S, Wittes J, Friedman L. Overview of results of randomized clinical trials in heart disease. II. Unstable angina, heart failure, primary prevention with aspirin, and risk factor modification. JAMA 1988;260(15):2259–63.
7. Muldoon MF, Manuck SB, Matthews KA. Lowering cholesterol concentrations and mortality: a quantitative review of primary prevention trials. BMJ 1990;301(6747):309–14.
8. Rose G, Blackburn H, Keys A, et al. Colon cancer and blood-cholesterol. Lancet 1974;1(7850): 181–3.
9. A co-operative trial in the primary prevention of ischaemic heart disease using clofibrate. Report from the Committee of Principal Investigators. Br Heart J 1978;40(10):1069–118.
10. Circulating cholesterol level and risk of death from cancer in men aged 40 to 69 years. Experience of an international collaborative group. JAMA 1982; 248(21):28539.
11. Anderson KM, Castelli WP, Levy D. Cholesterol and mortality. 30 years of follow-up from the Framingham study. JAMA 1987;257(16):2176–80.
12. Beaglehole R, Foulkes MA, Prior IA, et al. Cholesterol and mortality in New Zealand Maoris. Br Med J 1980;280(6210):285–7.
13. Cambien F, Ducimetiere P, Richard J. Total serum cholesterol and cancer mortality in a middle-aged male population. Am J Epidemiol 1980;112(3): 388–94.
14. Cowan LD, O'Connell DL, Criqui MH, et al. Cancer mortality and lipid and lipoprotein levels. Lipid Research Clinics Program Mortality Follow-up Study. Am J Epidemiol 1990;131(3):468–82.
15. Dyer AR, Stamler J, Paul O, et al. Serum cholesterol and risk of death from cancer and other causes in three Chicago epidemiological studies. J Chronic Dis 1981;34(6):249–60.
16. Farchi G, Menotti A, Conti S. Coronary risk factors and survival probability from coronary and other causes of death. Am J Epidemiol 1987;126(3): 400–8.
17. Garcia-Palmieri MR, Sorlie PD, Costas R Jr, et al. An apparent inverse relationship between serum cholesterol and cancer mortality in Puerto Rico. Am J Epidemiol 1981;114(1):29–40.
18. Gerhardsson M, Rosenqvist U, Ahlbom A, et al. Serum cholesterol and cancer–a retrospective case-control study. Int J Epidemiol 1986;15(2): 155–9.
19. Hiatt RA, Fireman BH. Serum cholesterol and the incidence of cancer in a large cohort. J Chronic Dis 1986;39(11):861–70.
20. Isles CG, Hole DJ, Gillis CR, et al. Plasma cholesterol, coronary heart disease, and cancer in the Renfrew and Paisley survey. BMJ 1989;298(6678): 920–4.

21. Iso H, Ikeda A, Inoue M, et al. Serum cholesterol levels in relation to the incidence of cancer: the JPHC study cohorts. Int J Cancer 2009;125(11): 2679–86.

22. Jancar J, Eastham RD, Carter G. Hypocholesterolaemia in cancer and other causes of death in the mentally handicapped. Br J Psychiatry 1984;145: 59–61.

23. Kagan A, McGee DL, Yano K, et al. Serum cholesterol and mortality in a Japanese-American population: the Honolulu Heart program. Am J Epidemiol 1981;114(1):11–20.

24. Kark JD, Smith AH, Hames CG. The relationship of serum cholesterol to the incidence of cancer in Evans County, Georgia. J Chronic Dis 1980;33(5): 311–32.

25. Keys A, Aravanis C, Blackburn H, et al. Serum cholesterol and cancer mortality in the Seven Countries Study. Am J Epidemiol 1985;121(6): 870–83.

26. Knekt P, Reunanen A, Aromaa A, et al. Serum cholesterol and risk of cancer in a cohort of 39,000 men and women. J Clin Epidemiol 1988; 41(6):519–30.

27. Kozarevic D, McGee D, Vojvodic N, et al. Serum cholesterol and mortality: the Yugoslavia Cardiovascular Disease Study. Am J Epidemiol 1981; 114(1):21–8.

28. Kromhout D, Bosschieter EB, Drijver M, et al. Serum cholesterol and 25-year incidence of and mortality from myocardial infarction and cancer. The Zutphen Study. Arch Intern Med 1988;148(5): 1051–5.

29. Menotti A, Keys A, Kromhout D, et al. All cause mortality and its determinants in middle aged men in Finland, The Netherlands, and Italy in a 25 year follow up. J Epidemiol Community Health 1991;45(2):125–30.

30. Menotti A, Kromhout D, Blackburn H, et al. Forty-year mortality from cardiovascular diseases and all causes of death in the US Railroad cohort of the Seven Countries Study. Eur J Epidemiol 2004; 19(5):417–24.

31. Morris DL, Borhani NO, Fitzsimons E, et al. Serum cholesterol and cancer in the Hypertension Detection and Follow-up Program. Cancer 1983;52(9): 1754–9.

32. Panagiotakos DB, Pitsavos C, Polychronopoulos E, et al. Total cholesterol and body mass index in relation to 40-year cancer mortality (the Corfu cohort of the seven countries study). Cancer Epidemiol Biomarkers Prev 2005;14(7):1797–801.

33. Pekkanen J, Nissinen A, Punsar S, et al. Short-and long-term association of serum cholesterol with mortality. The 25-year follow-up of the Finnish cohorts of the seven countries study. Am J Epidemiol 1992;135(11):1251–8.

34. Pekkanen J, Nissinen A, Vartiainen E, et al. Changes in serum cholesterol level and mortality: a 30-year follow-up. The Finnish cohorts of the seven countries study. Am J Epidemiol 1994; 139(2):155–65.

35. Peterson B, Trell E, Sternby NH. Low cholesterol level as risk factor for noncoronary death in middle-aged men. JAMA 1981;245(20):2056–7.

36. Peto R, Boreham J, Chen J, et al. Plasma cholesterol, coronary heart disease, and cancer. BMJ 1989;298(6682):1249.

37. Pocock SJ, Seed PT. Cholesterol in elderly women. Lancet 1992;339(8806):1426.

38. Salmond CE, Beaglehole R, Prior IA. Are low cholesterol values associated with excess mortality? Br Med J (Clin Res Ed) 1985;290(6466):422–4.

39. Salonen JT. Risk of cancer and death in relation to serum cholesterol. A longitudinal study in an eastern Finnish population with high overall cholesterol level. Am J Epidemiol 1982;116(4):622–30.

40. Schatzkin A, Hoover RN, Taylor PR, et al. Site-specific analysis of total serum cholesterol and incident cancer in the National Health and Nutrition Examination Survey I Epidemiologic Follow-up Study. Cancer Res 1988;48(2):452–8.

41. Schatzkin A, Hoover RN, Taylor PR, et al. Serum cholesterol and cancer in the NHANES I epidemiologic followup study. National Health and Nutrition Examination Survey. Lancet 1987;2(8554): 298–301.

42. Sharp SJ, Pocock SJ. Time trends in serum cholesterol before cancer death. Epidemiology 1997;8(2): 132–6.

43. Sharper AG, Phillips AN, Pocock SJ. Plasma cholesterol, coronary heart disease, and cancer. BMJ 1989;298:1381.

44. Sherwin RW, Wentworth DN, Cutler JA, et al. Serum cholesterol levels and cancer mortality in 361,662 men screened for the Multiple Risk Factor Intervention Trial. JAMA 1987;257(7):943–8.

45. Smith GD, Shipley MJ, Marmot MG, et al. Plasma cholesterol concentration and mortality. The Whitehall Study. JAMA 1992;267(1):70–6.

46. Sorlie PD, Feinleib M. The serum cholesterol-cancer relationship: an analysis of time trends in the Framingham Study. J Natl Cancer Inst 1982; 69(5):989–96.

47. Stemmermann GN, Chyou PH, Kagan A, et al. Serum cholesterol and mortality among Japanese-American men. The Honolulu (Hawaii) Heart Program. Arch Intern Med 1991;151(5):969–72.

48. Toshima H, Koga Y, Menotti A, et al. The seven countries study in Japan. Twenty-five-year experience in cardiovascular and all-causes deaths. Jpn Heart J 1995;36(2):179–89.

49. Tulinius H, Sigfusson N, Sigvaldason H, et al. Risk factors for malignant diseases: a cohort study on

a population of 22,946 Icelanders. Cancer Epidemiol Biomarkers Prev 1997;6(11):863–73.

50. Vartiainen E, Du DJ, Marks JS, et al. Mortality, cardiovascular risk factors, and diet in China, Finland, and the United States. Public Health Rep 1991;106(1):41–6.

51. Wald NJ, Thompson SG, Law MR, et al. Serum cholesterol and subsequent risk of cancer: results from the BUPA study. Br J Cancer 1989;59(6):936–8.

52. Westlund K, Nicolaysen R. Ten-year mortality and morbidity related to serum cholesterol. A follow-up of 3.751 men aged 40–49. Scand J Clin Lab Invest Suppl 1972;127:1–24.

53. Williams RR, Sorlie PD, Feinleib M, et al. Cancer incidence by levels of cholesterol. JAMA 1981; 245(3):247–52.

54. Wingard DL, Criqui MH, Holdbook MJ, et al. Plasma cholesterol and cancer morbidity and mortality in an adult community. J Chronic Dis 1984;37(5):401–6.

55. Yaari S, Goldbourt, Even-Zohar S, et al. Associations of serum high density lipoprotein and total cholesterol with total, cardiovascular, and cancer mortality in a 7-year prospective study of 10 000 men. Lancet 1981;1(8228):1011–5.

56. Chen Z, Keech A, Collins R, et al. Prolonged infection with hepatitis B virus and association between low blood cholesterol concentration and liver cancer. BMJ 1993;306(6882):890–4.

57. Chen Z, Peto R, Collins R, et al. Serum cholesterol concentration and coronary heart disease in population with low cholesterol concentrations. BMJ 1991;303(6797):276–82.

58. Schuit AJ, Van Dijk CE, Dekker JM, et al. Inverse association between serum total cholesterol and cancer mortality in Dutch civil servants. Am J Epidemiol 1993;137(9):966–76.

59. Tornberg SA, Holm LE, Carstensen JM, et al. Cancer incidence and cancer mortality in relation to serum cholesterol. J Natl Cancer Inst 1989;81(24):191721.

60. Petersson B, Trell E, Henningsen NC, et al. Risk factors for premature death in middle aged men. Br Med J (Clin Res Ed) 1984;288(6426):1264–8.

61. Feinleib M. Summary of a workshop on cholesterol and noncardiovascular disease mortality. Prev Med 1982;11(3):360–7.

62. Jacobs D, Blackburn H, Higgins M, et al. Report of the conference on low blood cholesterol: mortality associations. Circulation 1992;86(3):1046–60.

63. Baigent C, Keech A, Kearney PM, et al. Efficacy and safety of cholesterol-lowering treatment: prospective meta-analysis of data from 90,056 participants in 14 randomised trials of statins. Lancet 2005;366(9493):1267–78.

64. Browning DR, Martin RM. Statins and risk of cancer: a systematic review and metaanalysis. Int J Cancer 2007;120(4):833–43.

65. Dale KM, Coleman CI, Henyan NN, et al. Statins and cancer risk: a meta-analysis. JAMA 2006; 295(1):74–80.

66. Thompson MM, Garland C, Barrett-Connor E, et al. Heart disease risk factors, diabetes, and prostatic cancer in an adult community. Am J Epidemiol 1989;129(3):511–7.

67. Huxley R. The impact of modifiable risk factors on mortality from prostate cancer in populations of the Asia-Pacific region. Asian Pac J Cancer Prev 2007;8(2):199–205.

68. Platz EA, Clinton SK, Giovannucci E. Association between plasma cholesterol and prostate cancer in the PSA era. Int J Cancer 2008; 123(7):1693–8.

69. Platz EA, Till C, Goodman PJ, et al. Men with low serum cholesterol have a lower risk of high-grade prostate cancer in the placebo arm of the prostate cancer prevention trial. Cancer Epidemiol Biomarkers Prev 2009;18(11):2807–13.

70. Mondul AM, Clipp SL, Helzlsouer KJ, et al. Association between plasma total cholesterol concentration and incident prostate cancer in the CLUE II cohort. Cancer Causes Control 2010;21(1):61–8.

71. Batty GD, Kivimaki M, Clarke R, et al. Modifiable risk factors for prostate cancer mortality in London: forty years of follow-up in the Whitehall study. Cancer Causes Control 2011;22(2):311–8.

72. Solomon KR, Freeman MR. Do the cholesterol-lowering properties of statins affect cancer risk? Trends Endocrinol Metab 2008;19(4):113–21.

73. Solomon KR, Pelton K, Boucher K, et al. Ezetimibe is an inhibitor of tumor angiogenesis. Am J Pathol 2009;174(3):1017–26.

74. Zhuang L, Kim J, Adam RM, et al. Cholesterol targeting alters lipid raft composition and cell survival in prostate cancer cells and xenografts. J Clin Invest 2005;115(4):959–68.

75. Moyad MA. Heart healthy equals prostate healthy equals statins: the next cancer chemoprevention trial. Part I. Curr Opin Urol 2005;15(1):1–6.

76. Moyad MA, Merrick GS. Statins and cholesterol lowering after a cancer diagnosis: why not? Urol Oncol 2005;23(1):49–55.

77. Moyad MA, Merrick GS. Cholesterol, cholesterol lowering agents/statins, and urologic disease: part I–knowing your numbers. Urol Nurs 2006;26(2): 156–9.

78. Moyad MA, Merrick GS, Butler WM, et al. Statins, especially atorvastatin, may favorably influence clinical presentation and biochemical progression-free survival after brachytherapy for clinically localized prostate cancer. Urology 2005;66(6):1150–4.

79. Flick ED, Habel LA, Chan KA, et al. Statin use and risk of prostate cancer in the California Men's Health Study Cohort. Cancer Epidemiol Biomarkers Prev 2007;16(11):2218–25.

80. Friis S, Poulsen AH, Johnsen SP, et al. Cancer risk among statin users: a population-based cohort study. Int J Cancer 2005;114(4):643–7.

81. Graaf MR, Beiderbeck AB, Egberts AC, et al. The risk of cancer in users of statins. J Clin Oncol 2004;22(12):2388–94.

82. Jacobs EJ, Rodriguez C, Bain EB, et al. Cholesterol-lowering drugs and advanced prostate cancer incidence in a large U.S. cohort. Cancer Epidemiol Biomarkers Prev 2007;16(11):2213–7.

83. Murtola TJ, Tammela TL, Lahtela J, et al. Cholesterol-lowering drugs and prostate cancer risk: a population-based case-control study. Cancer Epidemiol Biomarkers Prev 2007;16(11):2226–32.

84. Platz EA, Leitzmann MF, Visvanathan K, et al. Statin drugs and risk of advanced prostate cancer. J Natl Cancer Inst 2006;98(24):1819–25.

85. Breau RH, Karnes RJ, Jacobson DJ, et al. The association between statin use and the diagnosis of prostate cancer in a population based cohort. J Urol 2010;184(2):494–9.

86. Gutt R, Tonlaar N, Kunnavakkam R, et al. Statin use and risk of prostate cancer recurrence in men treated with radiation therapy. J Clin Oncol 2010; 28(16):2653–9.

87. Murtola TJ. Statin use is associated with improved prostate cancer survival: is it time for a clinical trial? Expert Rev Anticancer Ther 2010;10(10):1563–7.

88. Randomised trial of cholesterol lowering in 4444 patients with coronary heart disease: the Scandinavian Simvastatin Survival Study (4S). Lancet 1994; 344(8934):1383–9.

89. Effect of simvastatin on coronary atheroma: the Multicentre Anti-Atheroma Study (MAAS). Lancet 1994;344(8923):633–8.

90. Prevention of cardiovascular events and death with pravastatin in patients with coronary heart disease and a broad range of initial cholesterol levels. The Long-Term Intervention with Pravastatin in Ischaemic Disease (LIPID) Study Group. N Engl J Med 1998;339(19):1349–57.

91. Results of the low-dose (20 mg) pravastatin GISSI Prevenzione trial in 4271 patients with recent myocardial infarction: do stopped trials contribute to overall knowledge? GISSI Prevenzione Investigators (Gruppo Italiano per lo Studio della Sopravvivenza nell'Infarto Miocardico). Ital Heart J 2000; 1(12):810–20.

92. Major outcomes in moderately hypercholesterolemic, hypertensive patients randomized to pravastatin vs usual care: The Antihypertensive and Lipid-Lowering Treatment to Prevent Heart Attack Trial (ALLHAT-LLT). JAMA 2002;288(23):2998–3007.

93. Long-term effectiveness and safety of pravastatin in 9014 patients with coronary heart disease and average cholesterol concentrations: the LIPID trial follow-up. Lancet 2002;359(9315):1379–87.

94. The effects of cholesterol lowering with simvastatin on cause-specific mortality and on cancer incidence in 20,536 high-risk people: a randomised placebo-controlled trial [ISRCTN48489393]. BMC Med 2005;3:6.

95. Beishuizen ED, van de Ree MA, Jukema JW, et al. Two-year statin therapy does not alter the progression of intima-media thickness in patients with type 2 diabetes without manifest cardiovascular disease. Diabetes Care 2004;27(12):2887–92.

96. Bestehorn HP, Rensing UF, Roskamm H, et al. The effect of simvastatin on progression of coronary artery disease. The Multicenter coronary Intervention Study (CIS). Eur Heart J 1997;18(2):226–34.

97. Blankenhorn DH, Azen SP, Kramsch DM, et al. Coronary angiographic changes with lovastatin therapy. The Monitored Atherosclerosis Regression Study (MARS). Ann Intern Med 1993;119(10):969–76.

98. Chonchol M, Cook T, Kjekshus J, et al. Simvastatin for secondary prevention of all-cause mortality and major coronary events in patients with mild chronic renal insufficiency. Am J Kidney Dis 2007;49(3): 373–82.

99. Colhoun HM, Betteridge DJ, Durrington PN, et al. Primary prevention of cardiovascular disease with atorvastatin in type 2 diabetes in the Collaborative Atorvastatin Diabetes Study (CARDS): multicentre randomised placebo-controlled trial. Lancet 2004; 364(9435):685–96.

100. Collins R, Peto R, Armitage J. The MRC/BHF Heart Protection Study: preliminary results. Int J Clin Pract 2002;56(1):53–6.

101. Crouse JR 3rd, Byington RP, Bond MG, et al. Pravastatin, Lipids, and Atherosclerosis in the Carotid Arteries (PLAC-II). Am J Cardiol 1995;75(7):455–9.

102. Crouse JR, Byington RP, Bond MG, et al. Pravastatin, lipids, and atherosclerosis in the carotid arteries: design features of a clinical trial with carotid atherosclerosis outcome. Control Clin Trials 1992;13(6):495–506.

103. Downs JR, Clearfield M, Tyroler HA, et al. Air Force/ Texas Coronary Atherosclerosis Prevention Study (AFCAPS/TEXCAPS): additional perspectives on tolerability of long-term treatment with lovastatin. Am J Cardiol 2001;87(9):1074–9.

104. Fellstrom BC, Jardine AG, Schmieder RE, et al. Rosuvastatin and cardiovascular events in patients undergoing hemodialysis. N Engl J Med 2009; 360(14):1395–407.

105. Ford I, Murray H, Packard CJ, et al. Long-term follow-up of the West of Scotland Coronary Prevention Study. N Engl J Med 2007;357(15):1477–86.

106. Furberg CD, Adams HP Jr, Applegate WB, et al. Effect of lovastatin on early carotid atherosclerosis and cardiovascular events. Asymptomatic Carotid Artery Progression Study (ACAPS) Research Group. Circulation 1994;90(4):1679–87.

107. Herd JA, Ballantyne CM, Farmer JA, et al. Effects of fluvastatin on coronary atherosclerosis in patients with mild to moderate cholesterol elevations (Lipoprotein and Coronary Atherosclerosis Study [LCAS]). Am J Cardiol 1997;80(3):278–86.

108. Holdaas H, Fellstrom B, Cole E, et al. Long-term cardiac outcomes in renal transplant recipients receiving fluvastatin: the ALERT extension study. Am J Transplant 2005;5(12):2929–36.

109. Holdaas H, Fellstrom B, Jardine AG, et al. Effect of fluvastatin on cardiac outcomes in renal transplant recipients: a multicentre, randomised, placebo-controlled trial. Lancet 2003;361(9374):2024–31.

110. Jukema JW, Bruschke AV, van Boven AJ, et al. Effects of lipid lowering by pravastatin on progression and regression of coronary artery disease in symptomatic men with normal to moderately elevated serum cholesterol levels. The Regression Growth Evaluation Statin Study (REGRESS). Circulation 1995;91(10):2528–40.

111. Kobashigawa JA, Katznelson S, Laks H, et al. Effect of pravastatin on outcomes after cardiac transplantation. N Engl J Med 1995;333(10):621–7.

112. Kobashigawa JA, Moriguchi JD, Laks H, et al. Ten-year follow-up of a randomized trial of pravastatin in heart transplant patients. J Heart Lung Transplant 2005;24(11):1736–40.

113. Koren MJ, Hunninghake DB. Clinical outcomes in managed-care patients with coronary heart disease treated aggressively in lipid-lowering disease management clinics: the alliance study. J Am Coll Cardiol 2004;44(9):1772–9.

114. Mercuri M, Bond MG, Sirtori CR, et al. Pravastatin reduces carotid intima-media thickness progression in an asymptomatic hypercholesterolemic Mediterranean population: the Carotid Atherosclerosis Italian Ultrasound Study. Am J Med 1996;101(6):627–34.

115. Mohler ER 3rd, Hiatt WR, Creager MA. Cholesterol reduction with atorvastatin improves walking distance in patients with peripheral arterial disease. Circulation 2003;108(12):1481–6.

116. Nakamura H, Arakawa K, Itakura H, et al. Primary prevention of cardiovascular disease with pravastatin in Japan (MEGA Study): a prospective randomised controlled trial. Lancet 2006;368(9542):1155–63.

117. Newman CB, Szarek M, Colhoun HM, et al. The safety and tolerability of atorvastatin 10 mg in the Collaborative Atorvastatin Diabetes Study (CARDS). Diab Vasc Dis Res 2008;5(3):177–83.

118. Pedersen TR, Wilhelmsen L, Faergeman O, et al. Follow-up study of patients randomized in the Scandinavian simvastatin survival study (4S) of cholesterol lowering. Am J Cardiol 2000;86(3):257–62.

119. Pitt B, Mancini GB, Ellis SG, et al. Pravastatin limitation of atherosclerosis in the coronary arteries (PLAC I): reduction in atherosclerosis progression and clinical events. PLAC I investigation. J Am Coll Cardiol 1995;26(5):1133–9.

120. Pitt B, Waters D, Brown WV, et al. Aggressive lipid-lowering therapy compared with angioplasty in stable coronary artery disease. Atorvastatin versus Revascularization Treatment Investigators. N Engl J Med 1999;341(2):70–6.

121. Sacks FM, Pfeffer MA, Moye LA, et al. The effect of pravastatin on coronary events after myocardial infarction in patients with average cholesterol levels. Cholesterol and Recurrent Events Trial investigators. N Engl J Med 1996;335(14):1001–9.

122. Salonen R, Nyssonen K, Porkkala-Sarataho E, et al. The Kuopio Atherosclerosis Prevention Study (KAPS): effect of pravastatin treatment on lipids, oxidation resistance of lipoproteins, and atherosclerotic progression. Am J Cardiol 1995;76(9):34C–9C.

123. Sato S, Ajiki W, Kobayashi T, et al. Pravastatin use and the five-year incidence of cancer in coronary heart disease patients: from the prevention of coronary sclerosis study. J Epidemiol 2006;16(5):201–6.

124. Serruys PW, de Feyter P, Macaya C, et al. Fluvastatin for prevention of cardiac events following successful first percutaneous coronary intervention: a randomized controlled trial. JAMA 2002;287(24):3215–22.

125. Serruys PW, Foley DP, Jackson G, et al. A randomized placebo-controlled trial of fluvastatin for prevention of restenosis after successful coronary balloon angioplasty; final results of the fluvastatin angiographic restenosis (FLARE) trial. Eur Heart J 1999;20(1):58–69.

126. Sever PS, Dahlof B, Poulter NR, et al. Prevention of coronary and stroke events with atorvastatin in hypertensive patients who have average or lower-than-average cholesterol concentrations, in the Anglo-Scandinavian Cardiac Outcomes Trial–Lipid Lowering Arm (ASCOT-LLA): a multicentre randomised controlled trial. Lancet 2003;361(9364):1149–58.

127. Shepherd J, Blauw GJ, Murphy MB, et al. Pravastatin in elderly individuals at risk of vascular disease (PROSPER): a randomised controlled trial. Lancet 2002;360(9346):1623–30.

128. Shepherd J, Cobbe SM, Ford I, et al. Prevention of coronary heart disease with pravastatin in men with hypercholesterolemia. West of Scotland Coronary Prevention Study Group. N Engl J Med 1995;333(20):1301–7.

129. Strandberg TE, Pyorala K, Cook TJ, et al. Mortality and incidence of cancer during 10-year follow-up of the Scandinavian Simvastatin Survival Study (4S). Lancet 2004;364(9436):771–7.

130. Teo KK, Burton JR, Buller CE, et al. Long-term effects of cholesterol lowering and

angiotensin-converting enzyme inhibition on coronary atherosclerosis: the Simvastatin/Enalapril Coronary Atherosclerosis Trial (SCAT). Circulation 2000;102(15):1748–54.

131. Wanner C, Krane V, Marz W, et al. Atorvastatin in patients with type 2 diabetes mellitus undergoing hemodialysis. N Engl J Med 2005;353(3):238–48.

132. Waters D, Higginson L, Gladstone P, et al. Effects of monotherapy with an HMG-CoA reductase inhibitor on the progression of coronary atherosclerosis as assessed by serial quantitative arteriography. The Canadian Coronary Atherosclerosis Intervention Trial. Circulation 1994;89(3):959–68.

133. Wenke K, Meiser B, Thiery J, et al. Simvastatin initiated early after heart transplantation: 8-year prospective experience. Circulation 2003;107(1): 93–7.

134. Wenke K, Meiser B, Thiery J, et al. Simvastatin reduces graft vessel disease and mortality after heart transplantation: a four-year randomized trial. Circulation 1997;96(5):1398–402.

135. Zanchetti A, Crepaldi G, Bond MG, et al. Different effects of antihypertensive regimens based on fosinopril or hydrochlorothiazide with or without lipid lowering by pravastatin on progression of asymptomatic carotid atherosclerosis: principal results of PHYLLIS–a randomized double-blind trial. Stroke 2004;35(12):2807–12.

136. Effects of pravastatin in patients with serum total cholesterol levels from 5.2 to 7.8 mmol/liter (200 to 300 mg/dl) plus two additional atherosclerotic risk factors. The Pravastatin Multinational Study Group for Cardiac Risk Patients. Am J Cardiol 1993;72(14):1031–7.

137. Freeman MR, Solomon KR, Moyad M. Statins and the risk of cancer. JAMA 2006;295(23):2720–1 [author reply: 2721–2].

138. Adam RM, Mukhopadhyay NK, Kim J, et al. Cholesterol sensitivity of endogenous and myristoylated Akt. Cancer Res 2007;67(13):6238–46.

139. Zhuang L, Lin J, Lu ML, et al. Cholesterol-rich lipid rafts mediate akt-regulated survival in prostate cancer cells. Cancer Res 2002;62(8):2227–31.

140. Di Vizio D, Solomon KR, Freeman MR. Cholesterol and cholesterol-rich membranes in prostate cancer: an update. Tumori 2008;94(5):633–9.

141. Freeman MR, Cinar B, Kim J, et al. Transit of hormonal and EGF receptor-dependent signals through cholesterol-rich membranes. Steroids 2007;72(2):210–7.

142. Freeman MR, Solomon KR. Cholesterol and prostate cancer. J Cell Biochem 2004;91(1):54–69.

143. Hager MH, Solomon KR, Freeman MR. The role of cholesterol in prostate cancer. Curr Opin Clin Nutr Metab Care 2006;9(4):379–85.

144. Harris WP, Mostaghel EA, Nelson PS, et al. Androgen deprivation therapy: progress in understanding mechanisms of resistance and optimizing androgen depletion. Nat Clin Pract Urol 2009;6(2):76–85.

145. Singer EA, Golijanin DJ, Messing EM. Androgen deprivation therapy for advanced prostate cancer: why does it fail and can its effects be prolonged? Can J Urol 2008;15(6):4381–7.

146. Singer EA, Golijanin DJ, Miyamoto H, et al. Androgen deprivation therapy for prostate cancer. Expert Opin Pharmacother 2008;9(2):211–28.

147. Huggins C, Hodges C. Studies on prostatic cancer: I. The effect of castration, of estrogen and of androgen injection on serum phosphatases in metastatic carcinoma of the prostate. Cancer Res 1941;1:293–7.

148. Fenton MA, Shuster TD, Fertig AM, et al. Functional characterization of mutant androgen receptors from androgen-independent prostate cancer. Clin Cancer Res 1997;3(8):1383–8.

149. Ross RW, Xie W, Regan MM, et al. Efficacy of androgen deprivation therapy (ADT) in patients with advanced prostate cancer: association between Gleason score, prostate-specific antigen level, and prior ADT exposure with duration of ADT effect. Cancer 2008;112(6):1247–53.

150. Taplin ME. Drug insight: role of the androgen receptor in the development and progression of prostate cancer. Nat Clin Pract Oncol 2007;4(4): 236–44.

151. Taplin ME, Balk SP. Androgen receptor: a key molecule in the progression of prostate cancer to hormone independence. J Cell Biochem 2004; 91(3):483–90.

152. Taplin ME, Bubley GJ, Ko YJ, et al. Selection for androgen receptor mutations in prostate cancers treated with androgen antagonist. Cancer Res 1999;59(11):2511–5.

153. Taplin ME, Bubley GJ, Shuster TD, et al. Mutation of the androgen-receptor gene in metastatic androgen-independent prostate cancer. N Engl J Med 1995;332(21):1393–8.

154. Taplin ME, Rajeshkumar B, Halabi S, et al. Androgen receptor mutations in androgen-independent prostate cancer: Cancer and Leukemia Group B Study 9663. J Clin Oncol 2003;21(14):2673–8.

155. Labrie F. Adrenal androgens and intracrinology. Semin Reprod Med 2004;22(4):299–309.

156. Veldscholte J, Ris-Stalpers C, Kuiper GG, et al. A mutation in the ligand binding domain of the androgen receptor of human LNCaP cells affects steroid binding characteristics and response to anti-androgens. Biochem Biophys Res Commun 1990;173(2):534–40.

157. Geller J, Albert J, Loza D. Steroid levels in cancer of the prostate–markers of tumour differentiation and adequacy of anti-androgen therapy. J Steroid Biochem 1979;11(1B):631–6.

158. Geller J, Albert J, Nachtsheim D, et al. Steroid levels in cancer of the prostate–markers of tumor

differentiation and adequacy of anti-androgen therapy. Prog Clin Biol Res 1979;33:103–11.

159. Belanger B, Belanger A, Labrie F, et al. Comparison of residual C-19 steroids in plasma and prostatic tissue of human, rat and guinea pig after castration: unique importance of extratesticular androgens in men. J Steroid Biochem 1989;32(5):695–8.

160. Shah S, Ryan C. Abiraterone acetate for castration resistant prostate cancer. Expert Opin Investig Drugs 2010;19(4):563–70.

161. Ang JE, Olmos D, de Bono JS. CYP17 blockade by abiraterone: further evidence for frequent continued hormone-dependence in castration-resistant prostate cancer. Br J Cancer 2009;100(5):671–5.

162. Scher HI, Logothetis C, Molina A, et al. Improved survival outcomes in clinically relevant patient subgroups from COU-AA-301, a phase III study of abiraterone acetate (AA) plus prednisone (P) in patients with metastatic castration-resistant prostate cancer (mCRPC) progressing after docetaxel-based chemotherapy. J Clin Oncol 2011;29(Suppl 7):4.

163. Antonarakis ES, Eisenberger MA. Is abiraterone acetate well tolerated and effective in the treatment of castration-resistant prostate cancer? Nat Clin Pract Oncol 2009;6(1):12–3.

164. Attard G, Reid AH, Yap TA, et al. Phase I clinical trial of a selective inhibitor of CYP17, abiraterone acetate, confirms that castration-resistant prostate cancer commonly remains hormone driven. J Clin Oncol 2008;26(28):4563–71.

165. Ryan CJ, Smith MR, Fong L, et al. Phase I clinical trial of the CYP17 inhibitor abiraterone acetate demonstrating clinical activity in patients with castration-resistant prostate cancer who received prior ketoconazole therapy. J Clin Oncol 2010;28(9):1481–8.

166. Danila DC, Morris MJ, de Bono JS, et al. Phase II multicenter study of abiraterone acetate plus prednisone therapy in patients with docetaxel-treated castration-resistant prostate cancer. J Clin Oncol 2010;28(9):1496–501.

167. Attard G, Reid AH, A'Hern R, et al. Selective inhibition of CYP17 with abiraterone acetate is highly active in the treatment of castration-resistant prostate cancer. J Clin Oncol 2009;27(23):3742–8.

168. Madan RA, Arlen PM. Abiraterone. Cougar Biotechnology. IDrugs 2006;9(1):4955.

169. Reid AH, Attard G, Danila DC, et al. Significant and sustained antitumor activity in post-docetaxel, castration-resistant prostate cancer with the CYP17 inhibitor abiraterone acetate. J Clin Oncol 2010;28(9):1489–95.

170. Forti G, Salerno R, Moneti G, et al. Three-month treatment with a long-acting gonadotropin-releasing hormone agonist of patients with benign prostatic hyperplasia: effects on tissue androgen concentration, 5 alpha-reductase activity and androgen receptor content. J Clin Endocrinol Metab 1989;68(2):461–8.

171. Mohler JL, Gregory CW, Ford OH 3rd, et al. The androgen axis in recurrent prostate cancer. Clin Cancer Res 2004;10(2):440–8.

172. Nishiyama T, Hashimoto Y, Takahashi K. The influence of androgen deprivation therapy on dihydrotestosterone levels in the prostatic tissue of patients with prostate cancer. Clin Cancer Res 2004;10(21):7121–6.

173. Montgomery RB, Mostaghel EA, Vessella R, et al. Maintenance of intratumoral androgens in metastatic prostate cancer: a mechanism for castration-resistant tumor growth. Cancer Res 2008;68(11):4447–54.

174. Mostaghel EA, Nelson PS. Intracrine androgen metabolism in prostate cancer progression: mechanisms of castration resistance and therapeutic implications. Best Pract Res Clin Endocrinol Metab 2008;22(2):243–58.

175. Titus MA, Schell MJ, Lih FB, et al. Testosterone and dihydrotestosterone tissue levels in recurrent prostate cancer. Clin Cancer Res 2005;11(13):4653–7.

176. Locke JA, Guns ES, Lubik AA, et al. Androgen levels increase by intratumoral de novo steroidogenesis during progression of castration-resistant prostate cancer. Cancer Res 2008;68(15):6407–15.

177. Dillard PR, Lin MF, Khan SA. Androgen-independent prostate cancer cells acquire the complete steroidogenic potential of synthesizing testosterone from cholesterol. Mol Cell Endocrinol 2008;295(1–2):115–20.

178. Fillios LC, Kaplan R, Martin RS, et al. Some aspects of the gonadal regulation of cholesterol metabolism. Am J Physiol 1958;193(1):47–51.

179. Haug A, Hostmark AT, Spydevold O, et al. Hypercholesterolaemia, hypotriacylglycerolaemia and increased lipoprotein lipase activity following orchidectomy in rats. Acta Endocrinol (Copenh) 1986;113(1):133–9.

180. Leblanc M, Belanger MC, Julien P, et al. Plasma lipoprotein profile in the male cynomolgus monkey under normal, hypogonadal, and combined androgen blockade conditions. J Clin Endocrinol Metab 2004;89(4):1849–57.

181. Pick R, Stamler J, Rodbard S, et al. Effects of testosterone and castration on cholesteremia and atherogenesis in chicks on high fat, high cholesterol diets. Circ Res 1959;7(2):202–4.

182. Leon CG, Locke JA, Adomat HH, et al. Alterations in cholesterol regulation contribute to the production of intratumoral androgens during progression to castration-resistant prostate cancer in a mouse xenograft model. Prostate 2010;70(4):390–400.

183. Heikkila M, Peltoketo H, Leppaluoto J, et al. Wnt-4 deficiency alters mouse adrenal cortex function, reducing aldosterone production. Endocrinology 2002;143(11):4358–65.

184. van Weerden WM, Bierings HG, van Steenbrugge GJ, et al. Adrenal glands of mouse and rat do not synthesize androgens. Life Sci 1992;50(12):857–61.

185. Spackman DH, Riley V. Corticosterone concentrations in the mouse. Science 1978;200(4337):87.

186. An S, Jang YS, Park JS, et al. Inhibition of acyl-coenzyme A:cholesterol acyltransferase stimulates cholesterol efflux from macrophages and stimulates farnesoid X receptor in hepatocytes. Exp Mol Med 2008;40(4):407–17.

What Do I Tell Patients About Saw Palmetto for Benign Prostatic Hyperplasia?

Christopher J. Kane, MD[a,b,*], Omer A. Raheem, MD[a,b],
Stephen Bent, MD[c], Andrew L. Avins, MD, MPH[d]

KEYWORDS

- Saw palmetto • Benign prostatic hyperplasia
- Lower urinary tract

HISTORY OF HERBAL THERAPIES FOR BENIGN PROSTATIC HYPERPLASIA

Historically, herbal therapy is considered to be the mainstay of complementary and alternative medicine for the treatment of benign prostatic hyperplasia (BPH).[1] Millions of people worldwide, including in the United States, use herbal agents to treat symptoms of BPH and prevent its progression.[2] Despite their widespread use for maintaining prostatic health in older men, the long-term efficacy and safety of over-the-counter phytotherapies for lower urinary tract symptoms (LUTS) attributable to BPH are not clear.

BPH is a common cause of morbidity among older men in the United States and other developed countries. Although BPH is a histologic process and its exact cause is unknown, this condition confers morbidity primarily through LUTS. Additionally, men with BPH, and particularly those with larger prostates as a result of BPH, are at an increased risk for complications, such as acute urinary retention, and may progress to requiring surgical treatment for BPH. In fact, although the availability of effective medical therapy has reduced the need for transurethral resection of the prostate (TURP), the traditional surgical treatment for BPH, the Centers for Disease Control's National Hospital Discharge Survey reports that 132,000 TURP procedures were performed in the United States in 2000. Although a working epidemiologic definition of symptomatic BPH is still being debated, the clinical manifestations of BPH are generally agreed upon. Clinical BPH, defined as an American Urological Association Symptom Index (AUASI) score greater than 7 (moderate to severe LUTS) and a depressed peak uroflow rate (<15 mL/s), affects 17% of men aged 50 to 59 years, 27% of men aged 60 to 69 years, and 35% of men aged 70 to 79 years.[3]

Men with bothersome LUTS caused by BPH can choose from a spectrum of traditional medical treatments, including alpha blockers and 5-alpha reductase inhibitors, minimally invasive therapies that use heat to damage or destroy prostate tissue, TURP, and other surgical therapies.[4] The Medical Treatment of Prostatic Symptoms trial tested finasteride and doxazosin, alone and in combination, for the prevention of BPH progression.[5] BPH progression was defined as a confirmed increase in an AUASI score by at least 4 points, acute urinary retention, incontinence, urinary tract infection or urosepsis, or new renal insufficiency. Almost all progression events were in the first 2 categories.

Disclosure: Dr Kane has received speaker honoraria from Aureon, Centocor Ortho Biotech, and AMGEN.
[a] Division of Urology, Department of Surgery, University of California San Diego, 200 West Arbor Drive, 8897, San Diego, CA 92103-8897, USA
[b] Urologic Cancer Unit, Moores UCSD Cancer Center, 3855 Health Sciences Drive, La Jolla, CA 92093, USA
[c] Department of Medicine, University of California San Francisco, San Francisco, CA, USA
[d] Kaiser Permanente, Northern California Division of Research, Oakland, CA, USA
* Corresponding author. Division of Urology, Department of Surgery, University of California San Diego, 200 West Arbor Drive, 8897, San Diego, CA 92103-8897.
E-mail address: ckane@ucsd.edu

Urol Clin N Am 38 (2011) 261–277
doi:10.1016/j.ucl.2011.04.005
0094-0143/11/$ – see front matter © 2011 Elsevier Inc. All rights reserved.

urologic.theclinics.com

Finasteride is a 5-alpha reductase inhibitor that blocks the conversion of testosterone to dihydro-testosterone, the major intraprostatic androgen, and reduces prostate size. Doxazosin blocks alpha-adrenergic receptors in the lower urinary tract, resulting in a reduction in smooth muscle tone in the prostate and bladder neck. Alpha-blockers rapidly improve voiding symptoms and urinary flow rate, and the improvements are long lasting. Common side effects are dizziness, retrograde ejaculation, and postural hypotension. The 5-alpha reductase inhibitors reduce prostate volume and decrease the risk of urinary retention and the need for surgical intervention. The reduction in prostate volume takes months. Common side effects are decreased ejaculate volume and, rarely, erectile dysfunction. For men with severe symptoms and large prostates, combination therapy was more effective than either therapy alone, but was associated with a greater risk of side effects and greater cost. Combination finasteride and doxazosin therapy is an attractive option, given the different mechanisms of action.[5]

Almost 30 phytotherapeutic compounds are currently available for the treatment of BPH. Those that have been studied most are extracts of the fruit of *Serenoa repens*, the saw palmetto dwarf palm that grows in the Southeastern United States. Second to saw palmetto is the extract of the bark of *Pygeum africanum*, the African plum tree.[6,7] The proposed mechanisms of action for saw palmetto include 5-alpha reductase inhibition, intraprostatic androgen receptor blockage, and adrenergic receptor antagonism, as well as an anti-inflammatory effect.[8] In vitro studies have shown that *Pygeum* extracts have antiinflammatory and immunomodulatory properties, effects on bladder contractility, modulation of androgen production, and direct effects on the function of prostate epithelium.[7,9] Although there is conflicting evidence in the literature concerning the efficacy and safety of saw palmetto in the treatment of men with LUTS secondary to BPH, a recent meta-analysis of saw palmetto conducted by the Cochrane Review committee concluded that there is no observed benefit of using saw palmetto in the treatment of LUTS related to BPH, compared with placebo.[10]

EVIDENCE OF CURRENT USE OF SAW PALMETTO AND OTHER HERBAL AGENTS IN TREATMENT OF BENIGN PROSTATIC HYPERPLASIA

The use of herbal therapies by adults in the United States has increased significantly in the last decade. It is estimated that 1 in every 5 people in the United States uses an herb to treat a condition or promote health.[11] Likewise, herbal therapy for BPH is rapidly gaining popularity in the Western world. A 2002 nationwide survey found that approximately 2.5 million men used saw palmetto for treatment of BPH in the United States.[1] It is estimated that up to 90% of patients newly diagnosed with BPH have already tried an herbal treatment by the time they were referred to a urologist.[2,12]

The trend in using phytotherapy for BPH can be partly explained by positive views of herbal therapies and personal values and beliefs.[13] However, the published literature raises concerns about the safety and efficacy of herbal treatments for BPH.[14]

Plant extracts are widely used by men with BPH in the United States and usually sold as dietary supplements. In Europe, these extracts are often prescription drugs.[15,16] A nationwide German study reported that 50% of urologists preferred saw palmetto over pharmaceutical agents for treatment of BPH.[17]

In a 2002 Cochrane meta-analysis of the effectiveness of saw palmetto extracts for men with BPH, 21 randomized trials 4 to 48 weeks in duration were identified, with 3193 total subjects. Data from the trials indicated that, compared with placebo, saw palmetto reduced nocturia by 0.76 times per night (10 trials), increased the odds of self-rated improvement 1.76 fold (6 trials), and improved peak flow rates by 1.86 mL/s (9 trials).[18] Adverse effects were mild and infrequent. Methodological problems noted within the trials included lack of standardized symptom scores and short study durations. The most common dosage was 160 mg twice daily, but a comparative trial showed similar effectiveness with the more convenient dosage of 320 mg once daily.[19]

There has been strong interest among numerous investigators, particularly urologists, to further examine the safety and efficacy of phytotherapy for BPH in the form of large multicenter clinical trials, such as the Complementary and Alternative Medicines for Urological Symptoms (CAMUS) trial. If the results of these ongoing clinical trials show effectiveness at reducing LUTS, men with BPH might find herbal therapy preferable to medical therapy because of the appeal of naturalistic herbal therapy and minimal side effects.

COLLECTION OF RELEVANT STUDIES FOR THIS REVIEW

The authors performed PubMed (www.pubmed.gov), Web of Science (www.isiwebofknowledge.com), and Cochrane library (www.cochrane.org) world literature searches for articles in the English language. The search terms saw palmetto and BPH or herbal agent and BPH returned 35 studies published between 2000 and 2011 worldwide. Nineteen randomized clinical trials (RCT) were identified, but only 8 RCT were included (≥100 patients) (**Table 1**); 4 meta-analysis studies (≥2 clinical studies) (**Table 2**), 7 experimental basic scientific studies, 2 prospective studies, and 3 retrospective studies (**Table 3**) were related to saw palmetto or herbs and BPH. Most of the world literature, in descending order, is from the United States,[9] United Kingdom,[4] Spain,[4] Germany,[4] Italy,[4] France,[4] Russia,[2] Romania,[1] Turkey,[1] Australia,[1] and Brazil.[1] All large RCTs and meta-analyses were carefully selected and reviewed.

THE CURRENT AVAILABLE HERBAL AGENTS USED IN THE TREATMENT OF BENIGN PROSTATIC HYPERPLASIA

Table 4 lists most currently available herbal agents, dosages, and adverse effects. The current published evidence of using saw palmetto and other herbal agents is briefly discussed next.

Saw Palmetto

The mechanism of saw palmetto is poorly defined. Investigators have proposed antiandrogenic activity via 5-alpha reductase inhibition and subsequent prevention of the conversion of testosterone to dihydrotestosterone,[7] an antiinflammatory effect,[16] competitive inhibition of androgen binding, decrease in the bioavailability of the sex hormone–binding globulin (SHBG),[15] and inhibition of growth factor–induced prostatic cell proliferation.[16,20,21]

In 2009, a detailed Cochrane Review analyzed 9 RCTs of saw palmetto with 2053 total patients. Five trials with 820 patients evaluated saw palmetto alone or combined with nettle root, beta-sitosterol, vitamin E, or tamsulosin versus placebo.[22–26] Four trials with 1233 participants evaluated saw palmetto alone versus control.[27–30] The most common commercialized extract of saw palmetto was Permixon (Pierre Fabre Médicament, Castres, France). The review concluded that saw palmetto was well tolerated but failed to improve urinary symptom score compared with placebo.[10]

A recent Italian study was conducted to evaluate the effect of saw palmetto in reducing intraoperative and postoperative complications of men undergoing surgical treatment (TURP or open prostatectomy) for BPH. The 114 patients were randomized to receive either pretreatment with saw palmetto or no pretreatment. No intraoperative complications occurred and no blood transfusions were required in the pretreatment group ($P<.001$). Additionally, the postoperative course was statistically significantly more favorable in the pretreatment group. This study suggests that pretreatment with saw palmetto before surgery for BPH is an effective measure for decreasing potential intraoperative and postoperative complications.[31]

Pygeum

Experimental studies have shown that Pygeum exerts an antiinflammatory effect, modulates androgen production, and decreases hypersensitivity of the detrusor muscle of the urinary bladder.[7,9] In a large European multicenter study, the effectiveness of Pygeum was examined against tamsulosin and finasteride in 2351 men with LUTS/BPH. Marked improvement of patients' urinary symptoms was observed in patients taking tamsulosin (68%) or finasteride (57%), but there was 43% improvement in patients who were on Pygeum.[32] In a meta-analysis of 2 studies, Mantovani[33] systematically examined the role of saw palmetto and Pygeum on patients with BPH. A total of 70 men participated in 2 studies. In the first study, patients were treated with 320 mg daily saw palmetto for 30 days. In the second study, patients received 320 mg of saw palmetto daily or 25 mg of Pygeum daily for 30 days. Both studies demonstrated marked improvement in urinary symptoms and prostate size, and general tolerability of the herbal agents.[33]

Nettle Root

Previous studies have shown that nettle root has antiinflammatory effects, binds to SHBG, and inhibits cellular proliferation. It also inhibits sodium-potassium ATPase action (Na-K ATPase).[24,34] The safety and efficacy of nettle root was investigated over a 96-week period in 219 men with moderate/severe LUTS caused by BPH.[35] Participants were randomized to receive a placebo or a fixed dose of 160 mg Sabal fruit extract combined with 120 mg nettle root extract (PRO 160/120) over 24 weeks, followed by another 24-week control period during which all participants received PRO 160/120. In the final 48-week follow-up period, all participants received PRO 160/120. International Prostatic Symptom Scores (IPSS), urinary flow rates, and residual urine volumes improved significantly in the treatment group, thus providing evidence of a clinically relevant benefit of using PRO 160/120 over a period of 96 weeks.[35]

PUMPKIN SEEDS

Pumpkin seeds are antihelmintic agents, but they decrease the binding capacity of androgen receptors to testosterone through competitive binding. They also have diuretic properties.[36] In

Table 1
Randomized clinical trials evaluating saw palmetto and other herbal agents in BPH

First Author	Year of Publication	Journal	Study	N	Main Findings/Conclusions
Anceschi	2010	Minerva Urol Nefro	RCT	114	This study suggests that pretreatment with saw palmetto before surgery for BPH is effective in reducing intraoperative and postoperative complications.
Bercovich	2010	Urologia	RCT	NA	A new plant extract (Pluvio), which contains avocado, soya oil and nettle root, was compared with controls in men with BPH. IPSS, uroflow, postvoid residual volume, prostate volume, and PSA were measured. This study showed that Pluvio is highly effective for the treatment of BPH.
Lee	2009	Clinical Trials	RCT/CAMUS	3300	This RCT is the largest to evaluate saw palmetto for the treatment of BPH to date and the only one to include a dose-ranging protocol. The results of this study will provide the most definitive test of the efficacy of saw palmetto in men with BPH.
Lopatkin	2007	Int Urol Nephrol	RCT	219	This study was designed to evaluate the safety and efficacy of a combined agent (160 mg *Sabal* fruit extract and 120 mg nettle root extract in men with BPH. IPSS was reduced by 53% (*P*<.001), peak and average urinary flow increased by 19% (*P*<.001), and residual urine volume decreased by 44% (*P* = .03). This study concludes that treatment with PRO 160/120 provides a clinically relevant benefit.
Bent	2006	NEJM	RCT/STEP	225	This study examined the role of saw palmetto in BPH treatment. No significant difference between the saw palmetto and placebo groups was identified over a 1-year period.
Hutchison	2006	Eur Urol	RCT/TRIUMPH	NA	Tamsulosin, finasteride, saw palmetto and *Pygeum* were all assessed in treating LUTS/BPH patients. Drug treatments were associated with some improvement compared with watchful waiting for most patients. Tamsulosin was the most effective in improving urinary symptoms (68%). Additionally, *Pygeum* therapy was shown to significantly improve urinary symptoms (43%).
Engelman	2006	Arzneimittelf-orschung	RCT	140	A combination of 160 mg *Sabal* fruit extract and 120 mg nettle root extract (PRO 160/120), compared with tamsulosin in treatment of BPH. Primary outcomes were IPSS and adverse events. The study supports noninferiority of PRO 160/120 in the treatment of LUTS caused by BPH.

Author	Year	Journal	Study type	N	Conclusion
Popa	2005	MMW Fortschr Med	RCT	NA	This study recommends the use of the combined *Sabal* extract and nettle root extract (PRO 160/120) in the treatment of BPH.
Zlotta	2005	Eur Urol	RCT	NA	This study compares saw palmetto, tamsulosin, and finasteride. After 3 months, there were no statistically significant differences between the 3 treatment groups in terms of IPSS and slight improvement in sexual performance. This study demonstrates that saw palmetto has no negative impact on male sexual function.
Debruyne	2004	Eur Urol	RCT/PERMAL	704	This study compares saw palmetto and tamsulosin for the treatment of BPH and concluded that 320 mg daily saw palmetto is slightly superior to 0.4 mg daily tamsulosin.
Willets	2003	BJUI	RCT	100	Saw palmetto was compared with placebo. This study concluded that there is no significant beneficial effect of saw palmetto over placebo.
Melo	2002	Int Braz J Urol	RCT	NA	This study analyzed the effect of combined *Pygeum* and nettle root extract, compared with placebo. This combination produced clinical and urodynamic effects similar to placebo.
Sökeland	2000	BJUI	RCT	431	This study compared combined *Sabal* and nettle root extract (PRO 160/120) to finasteride in patients with BPH. It showed that efficacy of both PRO 160/120 and finasteride was equivalent. Additionally, PRO 160/120 had better tolerability than finasteride.
Marks	2000	J Urol	RCT	44	This study compared the effects of saw palmetto to placebo and concluded that saw palmetto appears to be a safe, highly desirable option for men with BPH.
Glemain	2002	Prog Urol	RCT/OCOS	352	This study compared a combination of tamsulosin and saw palmetto with tamsulosin alone. It concluded that the addition of saw palmetto or tamsulosin did not provide any significant benefit.
Preuss	2001	Int Urol and Nephro	RCT	NA	This study examined the efficacy of a combination of rye grass, saw palmetto, beta-sitosterol, and vitamin E compared with placebo. After 3 months, the combined therapy had significantly lessened symptoms of BPH and no significant adverse side effects were noted.

Abbreviations: IPSS, International Prostatic Symptoms Score; NA, not available; OCOS, Omix contre Omix + *Serenoa repens*; STEP, Saw Palmetto Treatment of Enlarged Prostates; TRIUMPH, TransEuropean Research Into the Use of Management Policies for LUTS suggestive of BPH in Primary Health care.

Table 2
Meta-analysis evaluating saw palmetto and other herbal agents

First Author	Year of Publication	Journal	Study Design	Main Findings/Conclusions
Mantovani	2010	Minerva Urol Nefrol	Analysis of 2 studies	This meta-analysis concluded that a daily dose of 320 mg of saw palmetto can significantly reduce symptoms related to BPH with a good tolerability.
Tacklind	2010	Cochrane Database Sys Rev	Cochrane Reviews	This systematic meta-analysis showed that saw palmetto provides no improvement in urinary symptoms secondary to BPH, compared with placebo. Additionally, it found that saw palmetto was well tolerated.
Boyle	2004	BJUI	Meta-analysis	This meta-analysis showed significant improvement in LUTS and flow rate in patients treated with saw palmetto for BPH, compared with placebo.
Buck	2004	J Urol	Meta-analysis	This meta-analysis suggested a wide spectrum of activity of saw palmetto. However, the precise mechanism of action remained unclear. Balance and caution are needed when extrapolating the results of in vitro laboratory studies to the complex human situation.

a randomized study, the preparation curbicin, obtained from pumpkin seeds and dwarf palm plants (*Cucurbita pepo* and *Sabal serrulata*), was compared with a placebo in the treatment of BPH. A total of 53 patients participated, and after 3 months, urinary flow, micturition time, residual urine, and frequency of micturition significantly improved in the treatment group, indicating that pumpkin seeds were beneficial in treating BPH.[36]

African Wild Potato

African wild potato extract blocks the production of cyclooxygenase-1 (COX-1) and COX-2 prostaglandin biosynthesis. It also has antiinflammatory and free-radical scavenging activity.[37] Some specific African wild potato extracts, taken alone or in combination with other sources of beta-sitosterol, seem to reduce urinary symptoms and improve quality of life.[37,38]

Beta-sitosterol

Beta-sitosterol inhibits 5-alpha reductase enzyme activity and has potent antiproliferative effects on the prostate, possibly by inhibiting growth factors.[39,40] In vitro experimental studies have

shown the inhibitory effect of beta-sitosterol on multifunctional growth factors.[37,40]

Lycopene

Lycopene reduces proliferation of prostatic epithelial cells and improves urinary symptoms.[41] However, there is no strong published evidence to support the use of lycopene supplements to treat or prevent BPH. Previously published data have shown that increased consumption of tomato products and other lycopene-containing foods might reduce the occurrence or progression of prostate cancer.[42]

Red Clover

Studies of red clover in animal models have identified antiandrogenic and apoptosis effects on prostate cells.[43,44] However, there is no clear evidence that red clover reduces urinary symptoms in men with BPH.

Rye Grass Pollen

Rye grass pollen acts as an alpha-adrenergic receptor antagonist, is antiinflammatory, and inhibits prostate cancer cell growth. The most used extract of rye grass pollen is Cernilton. Some studies have reported decreased prostate size, improved urinary flow, and decreased residual urine volume in men treated for BPH with Cernilton.[45] Others reported no effect on objective BPH measures.[46] It is unknown whether or not rye grass pollen is comparable to finasteride or tamsulosin; however, it is comparable to *Pygeum*.[46]

Selenium

Selenium activates glutathione peroxidase, which reduces oxidative stress by handling free radicals and hydrogen peroxide. In addition, studies of selenium have reported contradictory evidence regarding its effect on prostate cancer risk. Population studies suggest that higher serum or toenail selenium levels are associated with a decreased risk of prostate cancer.[47] A recent Italian experimental study evaluated the antiinflammatory effects of saw palmetto, lycopene, selenium, and an association of the 3 on rat prostates. The saw palmetto-lycopene-selenium association caused a greater inhibitory effect on the expression of (COX)-2, indicating anti-BPH properties.[48]

Vitamin E

Research suggests that vitamin E might have an antiproliferative effect on benign hyperplasic prostate cells.[49] Several large RCTs provide conflicting evidence regarding vitamin E supplementation and prostate cancer.[50] The best evidence indicates that taking vitamin E supplements does not significantly reduce the risk of developing prostate cancer.[50]

Garlic

Garlic acts as a smooth muscle relaxant, and there is also preliminary evidence suggesting that garlic extract might help improve urinary flow, decrease urinary frequency, and reduce other symptoms associated with BPH and prostate cancer.[51] Additional preliminary evidence suggests that taking garlic supplements might decrease the risk of developing prostate cancer; however, the mechanism of action is unclear.[52]

Prickly Pear Cactus

Cactus acts as an antioxidant, and preliminary evidence suggests that some patients who take powdered prickly pear cactus flowers, 500 mg 3 times daily for 2 to 8 months, have subjective improvements in symptoms, such as urgency and feelings of fullness in the bladder.[53]

Saxifraga Stolonifera Meerb

This Chinese herb has been studied as a potential treatment for men with BPH.[54] A recent randomized trial compared the symptomatic effects on patients with BPH treated either with alpha blocker or *Saxifraga stolonifera* Meerb. Although this Chinese herb was effective in improving quality of life, prostate volume, and maximum uroflow rate for men with BPH, it was less effective than alpha blocker in improving IPSS.[54] Further studies are required to thoroughly investigate its potential role in treating men with BPH, with particular emphasis on its molecular basis.

Saireito

It is known that Saireito acts as a diuretic. A study of its efficacy in treating men with BPH has been reported.[55] Twelve men diagnosed with BPH who failed traditional medical therapy and still reported nocturnal frequency participated in the study. Nocturnal frequency decreased significantly and the results suggest that Saireito can be used as an effective treatment for nocturia in patients with BPH.[55]

Green Tea

Green tea and androgens are among the oldest medicinal agents used in traditional Chinese medicine. Epigallocatechin-3-gallate, a catechin in green tea, can modulate the production of androgens and other hormones. This property could be useful for treating hormone-related diseases, including BPH and androgen-dependent and androgen-independent prostate cancers.[56,57]

Fengweicao Granule

This Chinese herbal preparation is made from *Pteris multifida*. In a recent randomized trial, 108 patients with BPH received Fengweicao granule, and 47 BPH patients received finasteride. After 3 months, both groups had considerable improvement in IPSS, uroflow rates, and residual urine volumes, but no significant change in prostate volume was observed. The investigators concluded that Fengweicao granule has a positive effect in treating BPH.[58]

Ganoderma lucidum

Ganoderma lucidum is another Chinese herb proven to be effective in men with LUTS caused by BPH.[59]

Qianlie Sanyu

Qianlie sanyu is another Chinese herb proven to be effective in men with LUTS caused by BPH.[60]

Table 3
Other studies evaluating saw palmetto and other herbal agents

First Author	Year of Publication	Journal	Study Design	N	Main Findings/Conclusions
Bonvissuto	2011	Urology	Experimental	NA	A combination of lycopene, selenium and saw palmetto caused an inhibitory effect on prostate of rat. This association might be useful in the treatment of BPH.
Sinescu	2011	Urol Int	Prospective	120	Long-term treatment with 320 mg saw palmetto proved to be efficient in reducing urinary symptoms and improving sexual function in men with BPH.
Quiles	2011	Prostate	Experimental	6	This study suggests that *Pygeum* has an antiproliferative effect on prostate fibroblasts and myofibroblasts but not on smooth muscle cells.
Pais	2011	Adv Ther	Experimental	NA	A novel saw palmetto extract shown to effectively inhibit 5-alpha reductase enzyme activity that has been linked to BPH. This study confirms the effect of saw palmetto on prostate, compared with finasteride.
Agbabiaka	2009	Drug Saf	Retrospective	NA	This study evaluated the safety of saw palmetto and recommended higher quality reporting to improve safety assessments in the future.
Scholtysek	2009	Biochem Biophys Res Commun	Experimental	NA	This study showed the potential usage of saw palmetto and its extracts as antitumor agents.
Avins	2008	Compl Ther Med	Subanalysis	225	This study examined the safety and efficacy of saw palmetto in men with BPH. No significant differences were observed between saw palmetto versus placebo regarding adverse events.

Hizl	2007	Int Urol Nephrol	Prospective	60	This study evaluated the efficacy of saw palmetto alone versus tamsulosin and saw palmetto versus tamsulosin alone for patients with BPH. Both saw palmetto and tamsulosin seem to be effective in treating BPH.
Schleich	2006	Planta Med	Experimental	NA	This study compared the antiandrogenic activity of *Pygeum*, saw palmetto, and pumpkin seeds in treatment of BPH and prostate cancer. Results showed that *Pygeum* has the highest antiandrogenic effect and may provide a novel approach for the prevention and treatment of BPH and prostate cancer.
Habib	2004	Prostate Cancer and Prostatic Diseases	Comparative analysis	NA	This study indicated that sources of saw palmetto vary significantly between brands. It also evaluated the safety and efficacy of saw palmetto in BPH as well as its therapeutic benefits, compared with available medications.
Talpur	2003	Mol Cell Biochem	Experimental	NA	This study evaluated the antiandrogenic effects of saw palmetto and rye grass on prostatic enlargement in rats. Saw palmetto and rye grass influence prostatic hyperplasia via effects on androgen metabolism.
Vacherot	2003	Prostate	Experimental	NA	This study evaluated the role of saw palmetto as an antiandrogenic agent on human prostatic stroma and epithelium specimens obtained from men with BPH. Induction of apoptosis and inhibition of cell proliferation are likely the basis for the clinical efficacy of saw palmetto.

Abbreviation: NA, not available.

Table 4
Summary of currently available herbal agents for benign prostatic hyperplasia

Herb	Scientific Name	Family	Dosage	Adverse Effects
Antiandrogenic				
Saw palmetto	Serenoa repens	Arecaceae	Dried: 160 mg twice daily; Liquid: 0.6–1.5 mL or 0.5–1.0 g of berries in 150 mL of water 3 times daily	Nausea, vomiting, constipation, diarrhea, headache, hypertension, mild pruritus, decreased libido, and ejaculatory/erectile dysfunction
Antiproliferative				
Pygeum	Pygeum africanum	Rosaceae	Dried: 50 mg twice daily	Nausea, gastric pain, constipation, diarrhea, dizziness, headache, insomnia, restlessness, and visual disturbance
Nettle root	Urtica dioica	Urticaceae	Dried: 600–1200 mg daily Liquid: 1.5–7.5 mL daily	Mild gastric upset, allergic skin reactions, and sweating
Pumpkin seeds	Cucurbita pepo	Cucurbitaceae	Dried: 5 g twice daily	Potential electrolytes loss
African wild potato	Hypoxis hemerocallide	Hypoxidaceae	Dried: 60–130 mg divided into 2–3 doses daily	Nausea, vomiting, indigestion, diarrhea, constipation, anxiety, ventricular tachycardia, bone marrow suppression in patients with HIV disease, reduced absorption and blood levels of alpha- and beta-carotene and vitamin E
Beta-sitosterol	22,23-dihydrostigmasterol	Beta-sitosterol	Dried: 60–130 mg divided into 2–3 doses daily	Nausea, indigestion, diarrhea, constipation, erectile dysfunction, loss of libido, reduced absorption and blood levels of alpha- and beta-carotene and vitamin E
Lycopene	All-trans lycopene	Lycopene	Dried: 15 mg twice daily	Reduced plasma PSA level

Red Clover	Trifolium pratense	Fabaceae	Dried: 40–80 mg daily for 3 months	Rashlike reactions, myalgia, headache, nausea, and vaginal spotting; large amounts can induce bleeding
Antiinflammatory				
Rye grass pollen	Secale cereale	Poaceae	Dried: 126 mg 3 times daily	Nausea, abdominal distention and heartburn
Nutrients				
Selenium	Selenium	Selenium	For prostate cancer prevention, 200 mcg daily	Nausea, vomiting, abdominal pain, nail changes, fatigue, irritability, alopecia, and weight loss
Vitamin E	Alpha-tocopherol	Vitamin E	For prostate cancer prevention, 50–100 IU daily	Nausea, diarrhea, intestinal cramps, fatigue, weakness, headache, blurred vision, rash, gonadal dysfunction, and creatinuria
Miscellaneous				
Garlic	Allium sativum	Alliaceae	NA	Mouth/breath odor, gastrointestinal irritation, heartburn, flatulence, nausea, vomiting, and diarrhea
Prickly pear cactus	Opuntia ficus-indica	Cactaceae	Dried: 500 mg 3 times daily for 2–8 mo	Mild diarrhea, nausea, increased stool volume, abdominal fullness, and headache
Saxifraga stolonifera Meerb	saxifraga	Chinese herb	NA	NA
Saireito	Saireito	Chinese herb	Dried: 5.4 g daily	NA
Green tea	Green tea	NA	NA	NA
Fengweicao granule	Fengweicao	Pteris multifida	Dried: 5 g twice daily	NA
Ganoderma lucidum	Ganoderma	NA	Dried: 6 mg daily	NA
Qianlie Sanyu	Qianlie	NA	NA	NA
Bushenhuoxue	Bushenhuoxue	NA	NA	NA

Abbreviation: NA, not available.

Bushenhuoxue

Bushenhuoxue is another Chinese herb proven to be effective in men with LUTS caused by BPH.[61]

Saw Palmetto Treatment of the Enlarged Prostate Study

The Saw Palmetto Treatment of Enlarged Prostates (STEP) study was the first randomized, placebo-controlled trial of saw palmetto to be funded by the National Institutes of Health (NIH) and was designed to address the methodological weaknesses of earlier studies. Specifically, the STEP study initially convened an expert review panel from the National Center for Complementary and Alternative Medicine (NCCAM) to solicit and review applications from manufacturers of saw palmetto in an effort to identify and select the highest-quality product. The product selected for the trial was manufactured by Indena USA and was confirmed to have 92.1% total fatty acids and 0.33% total sterols, a standard that meets recommended guidelines from the US Pharmacopeia and other authorities on herbal products.[25] The study medication was produced in 1 batch to optimize consistency and was tested at the midpoint of the study and confirmed to have a consistent level of the proposed active ingredients.

Other methodological improvements in the STEP study included the relatively large sample size (225 participants), the long duration of follow-up (1 year), and the assessment of the adequacy of blinding. Earlier studies had not described the process of developing an adequately blinded placebo for saw palmetto, which has a bitter taste and a pungent odor. If participants in the treatment groups knew they were taking saw palmetto, then the observed benefits in earlier studies could have been at least partially caused by a placebo effect. In the STEP study, participants were asked at the end of the study which group they thought they had been assigned to, and a similar number in both groups thought they were taking saw palmetto (40% in the active group and 46% in the placebo group, $P = .38$), suggesting that blinding was effective.

Inclusion and exclusion criteria in the STEP study were set to be consistent with most prior, large, randomized controlled trials of pharmaceutical drugs for BPH. Men were older than 49 years and had moderate to severe symptoms (defined as an AUASI score of at least 8) and a peak urinary flow rate less than 15 mL/s. The study recruited 225 men and randomly assigned them to the same dosage of saw palmetto used in the vast majority of prior studies (160 mg twice daily). The STEP study had a high completion rate (96%)

and medication adherence rate (92% of study medication consumed), and the active and placebo groups showed no significant differences with respect to baseline characteristics.

The predefined primary outcome of the study showed that saw palmetto had no effect on urinary symptoms. As in most studies of BPH, there was a small decrease in symptom scores during the placebo run-in period. After that, the AUASI score decreased 0.68 points in the saw palmetto group versus 0.72 points in the placebo group (difference in change in AUASI scores between groups 0.04 points, 95% confidence interval −0.93 to 1.01). The lack of effect of saw palmetto can be visualized in **Fig. 1**, where the lines showing changes in symptom scores in the 2 groups almost overlap. The STEP study also found that saw palmetto had no effect on urinary flow rates. The rate of serious and nonserious adverse events was similar in both groups, providing some evidence that saw palmetto is safe. The STEP study provided compelling evidence that saw palmetto is not an effective treatment for BPH, and suggested that the positive results of some earlier studies may have been caused by their methodological weaknesses. One significant limitation of the STEP study was that it only assessed 1 dose of saw palmetto and, therefore, could not assess whether higher doses or a longer duration of treatment might produce beneficial effects. Consequently, the CAMUS study was designed to address the possibility that higher doses of this herb might produce beneficial effects.

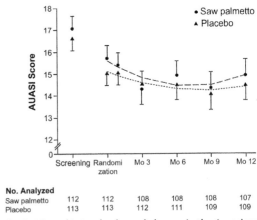

No. Analyzed					
Saw palmetto	112	112	108	108	108	107
Placebo	113	113	112	111	109	109

Fig. 1. Mean (±standard error) change in the American Urological Association Symptom Index (AUASI) scores in the saw palmetto and placebo groups. Values are screening represent prerandomization screening values. The full range of the scale is from 0 to 35, with higher numbers indicating more severe symptoms. (*Adapted from* Bent S, Kane C, Shinohara K, et al. Saw palmetto for benign prostatic hyperplasia. N Engl J Med 2006;354:557–66; with permission.)

The Complementary and Alternative Medicines for Urological Symptoms study

Among the many difficulties inherent in the study of phytotherapies is the choice of the product and the dose. Because part of the justification for studying phytotherapies is the perceived effectiveness of the supplement among large numbers of individuals who choose to self-medicate, it is important to replicate, as closely as possible, the actual conditions of use among the public. However, for many phytotherapies, there is great variation in the types of available products as well as the doses used. Hence, researchers are faced with difficult choices in conducting clinical studies and often have little theoretical or prior phase II work to guide the optimal choice of product to test.

Such was the case after the publication of the STEP trial of saw palmetto. Although the investigators chose a high-quality, well-characterized saw palmetto extract produced by an experienced European manufacturer, they were also aware that this extract was only one such product on the market and others were also widely used.[62] Second, the investigators chose to test the most commonly used dosage of saw palmetto, 320 mg/d (administered as 160 mg twice daily),[10] although higher doses have been used by men in the community. When the negative results of the STEP study were published, there were inevitable (and reasonable) concerns raised about the dose and product used in the trial and whether alternative products at higher doses might provide a demonstrable benefit. In addition, because it was a single-center trial, the generalizability of the results was of concern.

To address these concerns, the National Institute of Diabetes, Digestive, and Kidney Diseases, NCCAM, and the Office of Dietary Supplements jointly sponsored a large, multicenter, randomized double-blind clinical trial of 3 escalating doses of an alternative saw palmetto extract. This study, called the CAMUS trial, began enrollment in July 2008, with the intent of recruiting 369 men for an 18-month dose-escalation study (clinical trials.gov identifier # NCT00603304).

The CAMUS study was designed to specifically address areas of uncertainty raised by the STEP study. First, the investigators decided against a single dose of the extract in favor of a dose-ranging approach, starting with the widely used dosage of 320 mg/d (in a single dose for participant convenience), followed by a doubling, then tripling of the initial dose over the follow-up period. Second, because of the lipophilic nature of many of the extract's constituents, it was also felt that several months at each dose would be required to provide a fair test of efficacy; therefore, dose escalations were done at 6-month intervals. Third, the saw palmetto extract chosen was produced by an experienced manufacturer using an extraction technique (ethanolic extraction) different from the CO_2 extraction technique used to manufacture the product tested in the STEP study.

The inclusion criteria specified in the final protocol for the CAMUS required that participants be men aged at least 45 years, with an AUASI score between 8 and 24 and a peak urinary flow rate greater than 4 mL/s. Exclusion criteria were any prior procedure for BPH, taking a drug known to affect urinary function, serum creatinine greater than 2.0 mg/dL, evidence of liver dysfunction or coagulopathy (or anticoagulant use) at baseline, prostrate-specific antigen (PSA) greater than 10 ng/mL, urinary incontinence, cancer in the prior 5 years or cancer of the prostate or bladder at any time, neurologic condition affecting urinary function, and evidence of prostatitis or recurrent urinary tract infection. The primary outcome was change in the AUASI; secondary outcomes included participant global assessment of urinary function, the BPH Impact Index, peak uroflow, postresidual urine volume, PSA level, measurements of sexual and ejaculatory function, incontinence, perceived sleep quality, and the NIH Chronic Prostatitis Index. Assessments of symptomatic adverse events and detailed laboratory measurements were conducted at regular intervals.[63]

Recruitment for the CAMUS study was completed in April 2009 and the final participant was closed out in October 2010. Results of the trial are expected to be published in 2011. The CAMUS study is the largest placebo-controlled trial of saw palmetto to date and the only one to include a dose-ranging protocol.[10] The results of this study will provide the most definitive test of the efficacy of saw palmetto in men with LUTS and will likely have a major impact on future studies of botanic therapies for BPH as well as the clinical use of saw palmetto extracts.

SAFETY OF SAW PALMETTO EXTRACTS

Despite the large number of saw palmetto studies, there exist surprisingly little data on the safety of the extract. Most trials have not employed thorough methods for assessing potential adverse effects and few have conducted any laboratory assessments for subclinical toxicities. Most studies were of short duration (<3 months) and had small sample sizes. There are a small number of published case reports of adverse events potentially linked to the use of saw palmetto,[64–68] but most of these do not clearly establish saw palmetto as the causative agent.

The best data available on the safety of saw palmetto are from the STEP study.[25] As noted, the STEP trial included a large number of longitudinal laboratory measurements as well as regular, detailed assessments of symptomatic adverse events. A detailed analysis of the safety data from STEP has been published.[69]

Reassuringly, the examination of the STEP safety data revealed no evidence of clinically meaningful adverse effects attributable to saw palmetto. Although there were substantially more serious adverse events reported in participants randomized to placebo (18 in the placebo group vs 8 in the saw palmetto group), a large number of these occurred in a single individual, skewing the comparison. There was no significant difference in the percentage of participants in each treatment group who suffered at least 1 serious adverse event (5.4% in the active-treatment group vs 9.7% in the placebo group, $P = .31$) and most of these were not life threatening.[25,69]

Nonserious adverse events were approximately evenly distributed between the two treatment groups in STEP. The mean number of nonserious adverse events per person in the placebo and saw palmetto groups was 0.51 versus 0.47, respectively ($P = .72$). The proportion of participants experiencing at least 1 nonserious adverse event was also similar between the two groups (30.1% vs 34.8%, $P = .48$).[25,69]

Examination of the laboratory data from STEP was reassuring in that only a few significant differences between groups were observed, approximately the number that would be expected to arise by chance when conducting a large number of hypothesis tests; none of these differences were considered clinically meaningful. Importantly, there was no difference between the groups in changes in the levels of PSA over the course of the trial.[25,69]

Few other studies have reported comprehensive data on saw palmetto safety. One large study, a comparison of saw palmetto with tamsulosin among 704 participants over 1 year, found no effect on PSA levels over time.[27] Other studies have also found no effects of saw palmetto on PSA levels[25,26,70]; one small study (of biologic outcomes) did perform extensive laboratory testing on the trial participants and found no evidence of toxicity attributable to saw palmetto.[71] The most important data on saw palmetto safety will come from the CAMUS study, which has also included comprehensive adverse-event assessments as well as numerous longitudinal laboratory measurements.

A high-quality systematic review of potential adverse events associated with saw palmetto gathered data from the published literature; several governmental reporting agencies from North America, Europe, and Australia; saw palmetto manufacturers; and herbalist organizations.[72] The investigators found no firm evidence of toxicity associated with saw palmetto. The most commonly reported side effects were "abdominal pain, diarrhea, nausea, fatigue, headache, decreased libido and rhinitis."[72] However, the quality of the data was generally poor and no clear causal association with saw palmetto could be established, particularly because the rates of adverse events were similar in the saw palmetto and control groups among the comparative studies. No drug interactions were identified in this study or in a review specifically examining the potential for interactions between phytotherapies and prescription medications.[73]

On balance, saw palmetto appears to be quite safe, with no substantial toxicities noted in any studies. However, the generally small sample sizes of the studies do not provide sufficient statistical power to rule out the possibility of uncommon but serious toxicity. In addition, the duration of all of the studies were short in comparison to the many years that patients might be expected to use the supplement. The one exception is the effect of saw palmetto on PSA levels, for which substantial data show a lack of effect of the botanic on this parameter.

RECOMMENDATIONS

The best current evidence suggests that saw palmetto is no more effective than placebo in treating lower urinary tract symptoms caused by BPH. The CAMUS trial will determine whether higher doses of saw palmetto may be efficacious. Until the CAMUS results are reported the authors do not recommend saw palmetto for men with troublesome LUTS caused by BPH. However, the authors do not strongly discourage its use when men currently taking saw palmetto have confidence in its efficacy, because they may be enjoying a placebo effect and it does appear to be safe. There is no good clinical evidence that other herbal preparations are beneficial for men with LUTS caused by BPH.

REFERENCES

1. Barnes PM, Powell-Griner E, McFann K, et al. Complementary and alternative medicine use among adults: United States, 2002. Adv Data 2004;343:1–19.

2. Lowe FC, Fagelman E. Phytotherapy in the treatment of benign prostatic hyperplasia: an update. Urology 1999;53:671–8.

3. Jacobsen SJ, Girman CJ, Guess HA, et al. New diagnostic and treatment guidelines for benign prostatic hyperplasia: potential impact in the United States. Arch Intern Med 1995;155:477–81.

4. BPH Guideline Panel. Results of the treatment outcomes analyses. In: American Urological Association guideline: management of benign prostatic hyperplasia (BPH). Chapter 3. Available at: http://www.auanet.org/content/guidelines-and-quality-care/clinical-guidelines.cfm?sub=bph. Revised 2010. Accessed March 7, 2011.

5. McConnell JD, Roehrborn CG, Bautista OM, et al. The long-term effect of doxazosin, finasteride, and combination therapy on the clinical progression of benign prostatic hyperplasia. N Engl J Med 2003; 349:2387–98.

6. Fourcade RO, Theret N, Taieb C. Profile and management of patients treated for the first time for lower urinary tract symptoms/benign prostatic hyperplasia in four European countries. BJU Int 2008;101:1111–8.

7. Dedhia RC, McVary KT. Phytotherapy for lower urinary tract symptoms secondary to benign prostatic hyperplasia. J Urol 2008;179:2119–25.

8. Gerber GS. Saw palmetto for the treatment of men with lower urinary tract symptoms. J Urol 2000;163: 1408–12.

9. Ishani A, MacDonald R, Nelson D, et al. Pygeum africanum for the treatment of patients with benign prostatic hyperplasia: a systematic review and quantitative meta-analysis. Am J Med 2000;109:654–64.

10. Tacklind J, MacDonald R, Turks I, et al. Serenoa repens for benign prostatic hyperplasia. Cochrane Database Syst Rev 2009;15:CD001423.

11. Gardiner P, Graham R, Legedza AT, et al. Factors associated with herbal therapy use by adults in the United States. Altern Ther Health Med 2007;13:22–9.

12. Ernst E. Harmless herbs? A review of the recent literature. Am J Med 1998;104:170–8.

13. Astin JA. Why patients use alternative medicine: results of a national study. JAMA 1998;279:1548–53.

14. Speakman MJ. Who should be treated and how? Evidence-based medicine in symptomatic BPH. Eur Urol 1999;36(Suppl 3):40–51.

15. Di Silverio F, D'Eramo G, Lubrano C, et al. Evidence that Serenoa repens extract displays an antiestrogenic activity in prostatic tissue of benign prostatic hypertrophy patients. Eur Urol 1992;21:309–14.

16. Buck AC. Is there a scientific basis for the therapeutic effects of Serenoa repens in benign prostatic hyperplasia? Mechanisms of action. J Urol 2004; 172:1792–9.

17. Lowe FC, Ku JC. Phytotherapy in treatment of benign prostatic hyperplasia: a critical review. Urology 1996;48:12–20.

18. Wilt T, Ishani A, Mac Donald R. Serenoa repens for benign prostatic hyperplasia. Cochrane Database Syst Rev 2002;3:CD001423.

19. Stepanov VN, Siniakova LA, Sarrazin B, et al. Efficacy and tolerability of the lipidosterolic extract of Serenoa repens (Permixon) in benign prostatic hyperplasia: a double-blind comparison of two dosage regimens. Adv Ther 1999;16:231–41.

20. Vacherot F, Azzouz M, Gil-Diez-De-Medina S, et al. Induction of apoptosis and inhibition of cell proliferation by the lipido-sterolic extract of Serenoa repens (LSESr, Permixon) in benign prostatic hyperplasia. Prostate 2000;45:259–66.

21. Vela-Navarrete R, Escribano-Burgos M, Farré AL, et al. Serenoa repens treatment modifies bax/bcl-2 index expression and caspase-3 activity in prostatic tissue from patients with benign prostatic hyperplasia. J Urol 2005;173:507–10.

22. Preuss HG, Marcusen C, Regan J, et al. Randomized trial of a combination of natural products (cernitin, saw palmetto, B-sitosterol, vitamin E) on symptoms of benign prostatic hyperplasia (BPH). Int Urol Nephrol 2001;33:217–25.

23. Willetts KE, Clements MS, Champion S, et al. Serenoa repens extract for benign prostate hyperplasia: a randomized controlled trial. BJU Int 2003;92:267–70.

24. Lopatkin N, Sivkov A, Walther C, et al. Long-term efficacy and safety of a combination of sabal and Urtica extract for lower urinary tract symptoms— a placebo-controlled, double-blind, multicenter trial. World J Urol 2005;23:139–46.

25. Bent S, Kane C, Shinohara K, et al. Saw palmetto for benign prostatic hyperplasia. N Engl J Med 2006; 354:557–66.

26. Shi R, Xie Q, Gang X, et al. Effect of saw palmetto soft gel capsule on lower urinary tract symptoms associated with benign prostatic hyperplasia: a randomized trial in Shanghai, China. J Urol 2008;179:610–5.

27. Debruyne F, Koch G, Boyle P, et al. Comparison of a phytotherapeutic agent (Permixon) with an alpha-blocker (tamsulosin) in the treatment of benign prostatic hyperplasia: a 1-year randomized international study. Eur Urol 2002;41:497–506.

28. Glemain P, Coulange C, Billebaud T, et al. Tamsulosin with or without Serenoa repens in benign prostatic hyperplasia: the OCOS trial. Prog Urol 2002; 12:395–403.

29. Engelmann U, Walther C, Bondarenko B, et al. Efficacy and safety of a combination of sabal and Urtica extract in lower urinary tract symptoms: a randomized, double-blind study versus tamsulosin. Arzneimittelforschung 2006;56:222–9.

30. Hizli F, Uygur MC. A prospective study of the efficacy of Serenoa repens, tamsulosin, and Serenoa repens plus tamsulosin treatment for patients with benign prostate hyperplasia. Int Urol Nephrol 2007;39:879–86.

31. Anceschi R, Bisi M, Ghidini N, et al. *Serenoa repens* (Permixon) reduces intra- and postoperative complications of surgical treatments of benign prostatic hyperplasia. Minerva Urol Nefrol 2010;62:219–23.

32. Hutchison A, Farmer R, Verhamme K, et al. The efficacy of drugs for the treatment of LUTS/BPH, a study in 6 European countries. Eur Urol 2007;51:207–15.

33. Mantovani F. *Serenoa repens* in benign prostatic hypertrophy: analysis of 2 Italian studies. Minerva Urol Nefrol 2010;62:335–40.

34. Sokeland J. Combined *Sabal* and *Urtica* extract compared with finasteride in men with benign prostatic hyperplasia: analysis of prostate volume and therapeutic outcome. BJU Int 2000;86:439–42.

35. Lopatkin N, Sivkov A, Schläfke S, et al. Efficacy and safety of a combination of *Sabal* and *Urtica* extract in lower urinary tract symptoms—long-term follow-up of a placebo-controlled, double-blind, multicenter trial. Int Urol Nephrol 2007;39:1137–46.

36. Carbin BE, Larsson B, Lindahl O. Treatment of benign prostatic hyperplasia with phytosterols. Br J Urol 1990;66:639–41.

37. Berges RR, Windeler J, Trampisch HJ, et al. Randomised, placebo-controlled, double-blind clinical trial of beta-sitosterol in patients with benign prostatic hyperplasia. Lancet 1995;345:1529–32.

38. Klippel KF, Hiltl DM, Schipp B. A multicentric, placebo-controlled, double-blind clinical trial of beta-sitosterol (phytosterol) for the treatment of benign prostatic hyperplasia. Br J Urol 1997;80:427–32.

39. Cabeza M, Bratoeff E, Heuze I, et al. Effect of beta-sitosterol as inhibitor of 5 alpha-reductase in hamster prostate. Proc West Pharmacol Soc 2003; 46:153–5.

40. Kassen A, Berges R, Senge T. Effect of beta-sitosterol on transforming growth factor-beta-1 expression and translocation protein kinase C alpha in human prostate stromal cells in vitro. Eur Urol 2000;37:735–41.

41. Obermuller-Jevic UC, Olano-Martin E, Corbacho AM, et al. Lycopene inhibits the growth of normal human prostate epithelial cells in vitro. J Nutr 2003;133: 3356–60.

42. Gann PH, Ma J, Giovannucci E, et al. Lower prostate cancer risk in men with elevated plasma lycopene levels: results of a prospective analysis. Cancer Res 1999;59:1225–30.

43. Jarred RA, McPherson SJ, Jones ME, et al. Anti-androgenic action by red clover-derived dietary isoflavones reduces non-malignant prostate enlargement in aromatase knockout (ArKo) mice. Prostate 2003;56: 54–64.

44. Risbridger GP, Wang H, Frydenberg M, et al. The in vivo effect of red clover diet on ventral prostate growth in adult male mice. Reprod Fertil Dev 2001;13:325–9.

45. Buck AC, Cox R, Rees RW, et al. Treatment of outflow tract obstruction due to benign prostatic hyperplasia with the pollen extract, Cernilton: a double-blind, placebo-controlled study. Br J Urol 1990;66:398–404.

46. MacDonald R, Ishani A, Rutks I, et al. A systematic review of Cernilton for the treatment of benign prostatic hyperplasia. BJU Int 2000;85:836–41.

47. Yoshizawa K, Willett WC, Morris SJ, et al. Study of prediagnostic selenium level in toenails and the risk of advanced prostate cancer. J Natl Cancer Inst 1998;90:1219–24.

48. Bonvissuto G, Minutoli L, Morgia G, et al. Effect of Serenoa repens, lycopene, and selenium on pro-inflammatory phenotype activation: an in vitro and in vivo comparison study. Urology 2011;77:248. e9–16.

49. Wan XS, Zhou Z, Kennedy AR, et al. In vitro evaluation of chemopreventive agents using cultured human prostate epithelial cells. Oncol Rep 2003; 10:2009–14.

50. Heinonen OP, Albanes D, Virtamo J, et al. Prostate cancer and supplementation with alpha-tocopherol and beta-carotene: incidence and mortality in a controlled trial. J Natl Cancer Inst 1998;90: 440–6.

51. Durak I, Yilmaz E, Devrim E. Consumption of aqueous garlic extract leads to significant improvement in patients with benign prostate hyperplasia and prostate cancer. Nutr Res 2003;23:199–204.

52. Key TJ, Silcocks PB, Davey GK, et al. A case-control study of diet and prostate cancer. Br J Cancer 1997;76:678–87.

53. Jonas A, Rosenblat G, Krapf D, et al. Cactus flower extracts may prove beneficial in benign prostatic hyperplasia due to inhibition of 5alpha reductase activity, aromatase activity and lipid peroxidation. Urol Res 1998;26:265–70.

54. Li S, Lu A, Wang Y. Symptomatic comparison in efficacy on patients with benign prostatic hyperplasia treated with two therapeutic approaches. Complement Ther Med 2010;18:21–7.

55. Sugiyama T, Oonishi N, Onoe M, et al. Kampo preparations for prostatic hyperplasia: usefulness of Saireito for nocturia. Hinyokika Kiyo 2002;48:343–6 [in Japanese].

56. Liao S. The medicinal action of androgens and green tea epigallocatechin gallate. Hong Kong Med J 2001;7:369–74.

57. Hiipakka RA, Zhang HZ, Dai W, et al. Structure-activity relationships for inhibition of human 5alpha-reductases by polyphenols. Biochem Pharmacol 2002;63:1165–76.

58. Xue BX, Shan YX, Xiang G. Clinical evaluation on fengweicao granule in treating benign prostatic hyperplasia. Zhongguo Zhong X1 Yi Jie He Za Zhi 2008;28:456–8 [in Chinese].

59. Noguchi M, Kakuma T, Tomiyasu K, et al. Effect of an extract of *Ganoderma lucidum* in men with lower urinary tract symptoms: a double-blind, placebo-

controlled randomized and dose-ranging study. Asian J Androl 2008;10:651–8.

60. Xi JY, He JQ, Zhang X, et al. Observation of the therapeutic effect of qianlie sanyu capsule on benign prostatic hyperplasia. Zhonghua Nan Ke Xue 2005; 11:68–9 [in Chinese].

61. Wang L, Zhou S, Shao J, et al. System review of the Chinese medicine bushenhuoxue for treating benign prostatic hyperplasia. Zhonghua Nan Ke Xue 2004; 10:785–9 [in Chinese].

62. DiPaola RS, Morton RA. Proven and unproven therapy for benign prostatic hyperplasia. N Engl J Med 2006;354:632–4.

63. Lee JY, Andriole G, Avins A, et al. Redesigning a large-scale clinical trial in response to negative external trial results: The CAMUS study of phytotherapy for benign prostatic hyperplasia. Clin Trials 2009;6:628–36.

64. Hamid S, Rojter S, Vierling J. Protracted cholestatic hepatitis after the use of prostata. Ann Intern Med 1997;127:169–70.

65. Jibrin I, Erinle A, Saidi A, et al. Saw palmetto-induced pancreatitis. South Med J 2006;99:611–2.

66. Cheema P, El-Mefty O, Jazieh AR. Intraoperative haemorrhage associated with the use of extract of saw palmetto herb: a case report and review of literature. J Intern Med 2001;250:167–9.

67. Wargo KA, Allman E, Ibrahim F. A possible case of saw palmetto-induced pancreatitis. South Med J 2010;103:683–5.

68. Lapi F, Gallo E, Giocaliere E, et al. Acute liver damage due to Serenoa repens: a case report. Br J Clin Pharmacol 2010;69:558–60.

69. Avins AL, Bent S, Staccone S, et al. A detailed safety assessment of a saw palmetto extract. Complement Ther Med 2008;16:147–54.

70. Braeckman J. The extract of Serenoa repens in the treatment of benign prostatic hyperplasia: a multicenter open study. Curr Ther Res 1994;55:776–85.

71. Marks LS, Partin AW, Epstein JI, et al. Effects of a saw palmetto herbal blend in men with symptomatic benign prostatic hyperplasia. J Urol 2000;163: 1451–6.

72. Agbabiaka TB, Pittler MH, Wider B, et al. Serenoa repens (saw palmetto): a systematic review of adverse events. Drug Saf 2009;32:637–47.

73. Izzo AA, Ernst E. Interactions between herbal medicines and prescribed drugs: an updated systematic review. Drugs 2009;69:1777–98.

Quercetin for Chronic Prostatitis/Chronic Pelvic Pain Syndrome

Daniel A. Shoskes, MD[a],*, J. Curtis Nickel, MD[b]

KEYWORDS

- Prostatitis • Chronic pelvic pain syndrome • Quercetin
- Phytotherapy

The prostatitis syndromes are some of the most prevalent conditions in urology but also the most poorly understood. Although little controversy exists over the therapy for documented acute or chronic bacterial infections, most patients fall into the nonbacterial or prostatodynia group, now referred to as *chronic prostatitis/chronic pelvic pain syndrome* (CP/CPPS) or National Institutes of Health (NIH) category III. The origin, natural history, and appropriate therapy for these patients are unclear. Patient and physician dissatisfaction with these syndromes is high, making it an area ripe for patient interest in nontraditional and alternative therapies.

The polyphenolic bioflavonoid quercetin is a phytotherapeutic compound that has antiinflammatory and antioxidant properties. Its mechanism of action could be of value for several potential pathways in the origin of CP/CPPS. This article discusses the current understanding of CP/CPPS and how treatment with quercetin can be used alone or as part of multimodal therapy.

CLASSIFICATION

One of the earliest attempts at a classification system for chronic prostatitis was made in 1978 by Drach and colleagues[1] and was based on patient symptoms and localizing bacterial cultures published by Meares and Stamey[2] 10 years earlier.

The four-glass test localization study collected first-voided urine (VB1), mid-stream urine (VB2), prostatic fluid (expressed prostatic secretion [EPS]), and post–prostate massage urine (VB3), and subjected each to microscopic white blood cell (WBC) count and EPS. Acute bacterial prostatitis was defined as an acute febrile urinary tract infection (UTI). Chronic bacterial prostatitis was defined as recurrent UTI in which bacteria and WBCs were found in the EPS at levels significantly higher than any found in the premassage urine. The diagnosis of nonbacterial prostatitis was defined as WBCs but not bacteria in EPS or VB3. Finally, prostatodynia was used to refer to patients with typical symptoms but without any WBCs or bacteria recovered from prostatic secretions.

Unfortunately, this four-glass localization test was never formally validated as the basis for a classification system, and is seldom used by most physicians.[3] Still no evidence exists that men with no history of recurrent urinary tract infections but uropathogenic bacterial localized to the prostate experience a different response to therapy from similar patients with no uropathogenic localization. Traditional chronic bacterial prostatitis versus nonbacterial prostatitis responds differently to therapy. Recognizing this, a simpler two-glass test was popularized by Nickel and colleagues[4] as an adequate replacement of the more cumbersome four-glass test. In the two-glass test, only pre– and

Dr Shoskes and Dr Nickel are both consultants to Farr Laboratories. Dr Nickel is a consultant for Triton Pharma.
[a] Department of Urology, Glickman Urological and Kidney Institute, Cleveland Clinic, Desk Q10-1, 9500 Euclid Avenue, Cleveland, OH 44195, USA
[b] Department of Urology, Queen's University, Kingston General Hospital, 76 Stuart Street, Kingston, ON, Canada K7L 2V7
* Corresponding author.
E-mail address: dshoskes@mac.com

Urol Clin N Am 38 (2011) 279–284
doi:10.1016/j.ucl.2011.05.003
0094-0143/11/$ – see front matter

post–prostate massage urine is examined and cultured.

Recognizing the shortcomings of the current classification system, together with the lack of consensus for treatment, the National Institute of Diabetes and Digestive and Kidney Diseases began an initiative to address prostatitis in 1995. The NIH classification system was ultimately published in 1999.[5] Given the lack of understanding of the basic origin of CP/CPPS, the original etiology-driven classification system was replaced by a symptom/syndrome driven classification. Category I and category II are identical to the acute and chronic bacterial prostatitis of the previous system. Category III/CPPS is defined as the presence of genitourinary pain in the absence of uropathogenic bacterial. Category III was further divided into category IIIA and category IIIB. Category IIIA represents inflammatory CPPS in which WBCs can be found in semen, EPS, or urine after prostatic massage, whereas in category IIIB (noninflammatory CPPS), WBCs are not seen. Category IV, or asymptomatic prostatitis, includes patients without symptoms but for whom WBCs can be found in prostate secretions or in prostate tissue during an evaluation for other disorders (infertility, benign prostate hyperplasia, or prostate cancer). The new classification system has been validated for both research and clinical practice.[6]

CATEGORY III (CPPS)

CPPS is both the most common form of prostatitis and the most cryptic. The most common symptom is pain, which may be felt in the lower abdomen, pelvis, perineum, or genitals. Urinary complaints are common and may include both voiding and storage symptoms. Additionally, many complain of erectile dysfunction and ejaculatory pain. CP/CPPS is a significant health problem. Prevalence is between 2% and 16%, depending on the population studied, the epidemiologic method, and the definitions of prostatitis. This prevalence reflects a significant burden on the health system, wherein prostatitis is diagnosed in two million physician visits annually.[7] Furthermore, its financial impact is not negligible, with direct medical costs estimated at $6500 per year per person.[8]

The origin and pathophysiology are controversial, and in fact the disorder likely represents different underlying origins which produce a common symptom complex. Some patients with CPPS may have a true bacterial infection. Detection may be missed because cultures are not properly performed,[9] difficult-to-culture organisms are not searched for (eg, ureaplasma, mycoplasma), or the bacteria may not be identifiable using current culture techniques.[10] In the absence of infection, evidence shows an inflammatory or autoimmune component to CPPS. Even in the absence of visible WBCs, EPS and semen of men with CPPS have elevated levels of inflammatory cytokine[11] and oxidative stress.[12] Furthermore, symptomatic response to antibiotics in patients with CPPS may be from direct antiinflammatory rather than antimicrobial effects of these drugs.[13] Finally, much of the pain of CPPS is likely related to pelvic muscle spasm, which may be secondary to infective or inflammatory conditions mentioned earlier, or may be the primary problem in the absence of any prostatic pathology.[14] Pelvic muscle spasm can lead to chronic intermittent hypoxia, which may be improved by antioxidant therapy.[15]

CLINICAL PHENOTYPING OF CPPS

The authors believe that the only rational approach to patients with these disparate mechanisms and symptoms is to develop a phenotype that is clinically meaningful and, most importantly, that can drive and improve therapy. In response to this need, the UPOINT phenotyping classification system was recently developed for patients diagnosed with chronic pelvic pain.[16] UPOINT is a six-point clinical classification system that categorizes patients into six clinically identifiable domains: urinary, psychosocial, organ-specific, infection, neurologic/systemic, and tenderness of skeletal muscle. This clinical classification system is not necessarily based on etiology (but may be eventually) and remains flexible (can incorporate new epidemiology, therapeutic, and biomarker research as it becomes available). The key features of each domain are that they may be scored as positive or negative based on simple clinical criteria, they are discriminative in the populations of interest (ie, it would be of no value if almost all patients fell into a very few phenotypes), and each is associated with specific therapies with at least some reasonable evidence for efficacy. Because mulitmodal therapy is superior to unimodal or stepwise therapy in men[17] and women[18] with pelvic pain, the UPOINT phenotype provides a framework for rational multiple treatment selection.

The authors and others[19–23] have now studied the UPOINT system in men with category III prostatitis (CPPS). These studies retrospectively evaluated patients with these diagnoses and classified their phenotype as a yes/no for each of the six domains in **Box 1**.

In 90 men with CPPS the authors found that the percentage of patients with positive responses in each domain was urinary, 52%; psychosocial,

Box 1
The six domains of the UPOINT system

1. Urinary
   Patient complaint of bothersome urgency, frequency, or nocturia
   Post-void residual >100 mL
   Obstructive voiding symptoms (or maximum flow rate <15 mL/s)
2. Psychosocial
   Clinical depression
   Evidence of catastrophizing (helplessness, hopelessness)
3. Organ-specific
   Representative tenderness on light palpation of prostate
   Leukocytosis in prostatic fluid
   Hematospermia
4. Infection
   Exclude patients with clinical cystitis or bacterial prostatitis (includes past history of documented UTI associated with initiation or flare)
   Atypical bacteria in urine or positive prostatic fluid cultures in absence of UTI
5. Neurologic/systemic conditions
   Pain beyond abdomen and pelvis
   Irritable bowel syndrome
   Fibromyalgia
   Chronic fatigue syndrome
6. Tenderness of skeletal muscles
   Palpable muscle spasm or myofascial painful trigger points in abdomen and pelvic floor

34%; organ-specific, 61%; infection, 16%; neurologic/systemic, 37%; and tenderness, 53%. A significant stepwise increase in total symptom severity occurred as the number of positive domains increased.[20] Other investigators have subsequently replicated these initial observations.[19,23]

QUERCETIN: AN ANTIINFLAMMATORY AND ANTIOXIDANT NUTRACEUTICAL

The bioflavonoids are a family of polyphenolic molecules found in a variety of plants that have significant antioxidant and antiinflammatory properties. Quercetin is a member of this family found in red wine, green tea, and onions (**Fig. 1**). It is a potent free oxygen scavenger,[24] antioxidant,[25] and antiinflammatory agent.[26] It reduces inflammation through inhibiting the production of cytokines such as interleukin (IL)-6,[27] IL-8,[28] and tumor necrosis factor[29] by inhibiting the promoter nuclear factor κB (NF-κB).[30] These cytokines are elevated in the semen and prostate fluid of men with CPPS.[31] Furthermore, in an animal model of inflammatory pain, quercetin reduced pain, oxidative stress, and cytokine production.[32] Absorption of dietary quercetin is variable and dependent on gut flora.[33]

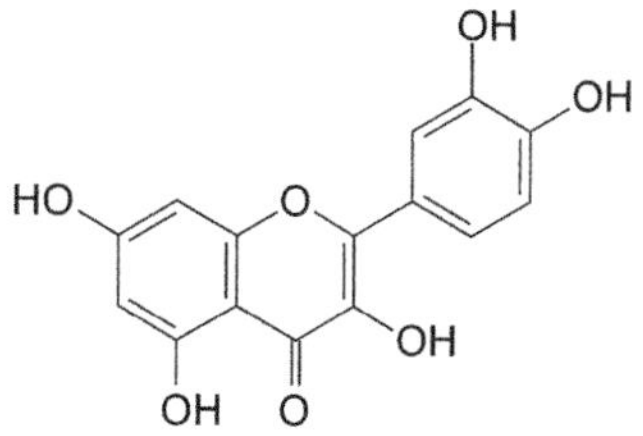

Fig. 1. Chemical structure of quercetin.

Quercetin has been studied in humans both for epidemiologic links between consumption and disease and for direct interventions through increased intake. In the Zutphen Elderly study, higher dietary quercetin intake was associated with decreased risk of cardiac disease.[34] In a British case-control study, increased quercetin intake was associated with reduced risk of developing colon cancer.[35] A case-control study in New York state found reduced prostate cancer risk among men with the highest quercetin intake compared with those with the lowest.[36] Treatment studies have focused on inflammation and cancer. A prospective controlled study found topical quercetin accelerates the healing of aphthous mouth ulcers.[37] Oral quercetin supplementation raises plasma quercetin levels in normal volunteers.[38] Six weeks of quercetin therapy reduced systolic blood pressure and oxidized low-density lipoprotein in overweight adults.[39] A combination of quercetin and curcumin reduced the number and size of ileal and rectal adenomas in patients with familial adenomatous polyposis.[40] Finally, a combination of quercetin and curcumin improved early graft function in recipients of deceased donor kidney transplants.[41]

Quercetin has theoretical benefits for patients with an ongoing inflammatory or ischemic process, which may underlie CPPS. In addition, because patients with CPPS often avoid foods rich in flavonoids (green tea [caffeine], red wine [alcohol]), they may have an actual dietary deficiency of quercetin. An initial prospective, double-blind, placebo-controlled trial of 500 mg of quercetin administered twice daily for 4 weeks was done using the National Institutes of Health Chronic Prostatitis Symptoms Index (NIH-CPSI) as the primary end point.[42] Patients taking placebo had a mean improvement in NIH-CPSI from 20.2 to 18.8, and those taking quercetin had a mean improvement from 21.0 to 13.1 (P = .003). At least a 25% improvement of symptoms was seen in 20% of patients taking placebo and 67% of those taking the bioflavonoid. This 25% threshold is associated with patient perception of improvement after therapy. A third group of patients received Prosta-Q (Farr Labs, Beverly Hills, CA, USA), a commercial formulation containing quercetin with bromelain and papain, which are digestive enzymes known to increase the intestinal absorption of quercetin. In this group, 82% of the patients showed a significant improvement of symptoms.

Several mechanisms may contribute to the beneficial effects of quercetin in CPPS. CPPS is associated with elevated oxidative stress in EPS and semen,[43] and patients who experience improvement with quercetin have a reduction in oxidative stress metabolite F2-isoprostane in their EPS.[42] Furthermore, quercetin therapy reduces inflammation as measured by prostaglandin E2 levels in EPS, and increases the levels of prostatic β-endorphins.[44] To explain why some patients experience response to quercetin therapy whereas others do not, blood from patients with CPPS treated with quercetin was analyzed for cytokine polymorphisms. Of the 28 patients treated with the antiinflammatory quercetin, all 11 in whom treatment had failed had the low tumor necrosis factor genotype versus 29.4% of those in whom treatment succeeded (P = .0003). Similarly men with quercetin treatment failure were much less likely to have the low IL-10 genotype than those with treatment success (9.1% vs 47.1%; P = .04). Therefore, men with a "low inflammation" phenotype were less likely to improve with quercetin. Finally, quercetin has weak antibacterial and antifungal properties that might conceivably play a role in CPPS.[45]

Side effects with quercetin therapy are rare. Some patients experience nausea if taking it on an empty stomach. Some patients have reported transient joint pain when quercetin is taken at high doses. Orange pigment in some preparations may show up in semen, and patients can be reassured that this is caused by the dye and not an infection. Because quercetin binds to the DNA gyrase site on Escherichia coli, where quinolone antibiotics bind, quercetin could theoretically interfere with quinolone antibiotics, and therefore the two should not be used together.[46] Quercetin may, however, be safely combined with nonquinolone antibiotics.

ROLE OF QUERCETIN IN CPPS THERAPY

Multimodal therapy for CPPS has advantages given the syndrome's heterogeneity, and the authors believe that the best results can be obtained through targeting therapy using the UPOINT phenotype system. They have focused on using quercetin primarily for patients with the organ-specific domain, whether the evidence for organ involvement comes from the bladder or prostate. In a prospective study of 100 men with CPPS treated according to the UPOINT phenotype, 84% had significant improvement in symptoms with a minimum follow-up of 6 months.[47] In this study, 70% were positive for the organ-specific domain and received either quercetin alone (Prosta-Q, Farr Laboratories, Los Angeles, CA, USA) or quercetin in combination with pollen extract (Q-Urol, Farr Laboratories). In the group as a whole, a treatment regimen that included quercetin had the strongest impact on symptom improvement.

Whether quercetin may have other beneficial effects in patients with CPPS is not proven. Given the relationship between prostatic inflammation and prostate cancer risk, and quercetin's ability to inhibit prostate cancer cells in vitro, a potential role in prostate cancer prevention is possible. Furthermore, the increased self-reported incidence of cardiovascular disease in men with CPPS[48] suggests that quercetin's reduction in cardiac event risk may be another potential benefit. The authors recently observed improvement in peripheral arterial tone in patients with CPPS who were treated with quercetin.[49]

The authors typically prescribe quercetin at 500 mg two to three times per day, preferably taken with food. Some patients note improvement in symptoms within days, but the authors recommend at least a 6-week trial. If improvement begins within 6 weeks, symptoms usually continue to improve further up to 3 months. The authors often combine quercetin with bromelain and papain to help enhance absorption using the same specific dietary supplements from their successful past prospective clinical studies.[42,47] As part of their planned multimodal therapy plan, they use a rationale of adding another potentially effective phytotherapeutic agent, pollen extract preparation (see article on Cernilton elsewhere in this issue), for patients with an organ-specific clinical phenotype. However, as with all multimodal strategies, no evidence from randomized placebo-controlled trials confirms the efficacy of the wide variety of combinations available for these patients. The authors caution against quercetin preparations that contain high doses of vitamin C, which can acidify the urine and potentially worsen symptoms. They also caution against the theoretical interaction with quinolone antibiotics and suggest that quercetin be held during quinolone therapy. Quercetin is an important component of a multimodal therapeutic program directed by the UPOINT phenotype presentation by each individual patient.

SUMMARY

Quercetin is a polyphenolic bioflavonoid that may benefit men with CPPS through antiinflammatory and antioxidant mechanisms. It may be best indicated for patients with CPPS whose UPOINT phenotype includes the organ-specific domain, as part of a directed multimodal therapeutic strategy.

REFERENCES

1. Drach GW, Fair WR, Meares EM, et al. Classification of benign diseases associated with prostatic pain: prostatitis or prostatodynia? J Urol 1978;120(2):266.
2. Meares EM, Stamey TA. Bacteriologic localization patterns in bacterial prostatitis and urethritis. Invest Urol 1968;5:492–518.
3. Kiyota H, Onodera S, Ohishi Y, et al. Questionnaire survey of Japanese urologists concerning the diagnosis and treatment of chronic prostatitis and chronic pelvic pain syndrome. Int J Urol 2003;10: 636–42.
4. Nickel JC, Shoskes D, Wang Y, et al. How does the pre-massage and post-massage 2-glass test compare to the Meares-Stamey 4-glass test in men with chronic prostatitis/chronic pelvic pain syndrome? J Urol 2006;176:119–24.
5. Krieger JN, Nyberg LJ, Nickel JC. NIH consensus definition and classification of prostatitis. JAMA 1999;282(3):236–7.
6. Nickel JC, Nyberg LM, Hennenfent M. Research guidelines for chronic prostatitis: consensus report from the first National Institutes of Health International Prostatitis Collaborative Network. Urology 1999;54:229–33.
7. Turner JA, Ciol MA, Von Korff M, et al. Healthcare use and costs of primary and secondary care patients with prostatitis. Urology 2004;63:1031–5.
8. Clemens JQ, Markossian T, Calhoun EA. Comparison of economic impact of chronic prostatitis/chronic pelvic pain syndrome and interstitial cystitis/painful bladder syndrome. Urology 2009; 73:743–6.
9. McNaughton Collins M, Fowler FJJ, Elliott DB, et al. Diagnosing and treating chronic prostatitis: do urologists use the four-glass test? Urology 2000;55:403–7.
10. Shoskes DA, Shahed AR. Detection of bacterial signal by 16S rRNA polymerase chain reaction in expressed prostatic secretions predicts response to antibiotic therapy in men with chronic pelvic pain syndrome. Tech Urol 2000;6:240–2.
11. John H, Maake C, Barghorn A, et al. Immunological alterations in the ejaculate of chronic prostatitis patients: clues for autoimmunity. Andrologia 2003; 35:294–9.
12. Shahed AR, Shoskes DA. Correlation of beta-endorphin and prostaglandin E2 levels in prostatic fluid of patients with chronic prostatitis with diagnosis and treatment response. J Urol 2001;166: 1738–41.
13. Basyigit I, Yildiz F, Ozkara SK, et al. The effect of clarithromycin on inflammatory markers in chronic obstructive pulmonary disease: preliminary data. Ann Pharmacother 2004;38:1400–5.
14. Westesson KE, Shoskes DA. Chronic prostatitis/chronic pelvic pain syndrome and pelvic floor spasm: can we diagnose and treat? Curr Urol Rep 2010;11:261–4.
15. Phillips SA, Olson EB, Lombard JH, et al. Chronic intermittent hypoxia alters NE reactivity and mechanics of skeletal muscle resistance arteries. J Appl Physiol 2006;100:1117–23.
16. Shoskes DA, Nickel JC, Rackley RR, et al. Clinical phenotyping in chronic prostatitis/chronic pelvic pain syndrome and interstitial cystitis: a management strategy for urologic chronic pelvic pain syndromes. Prostate Cancer Prostatic Dis 2009;12:177–83.
17. Shoskes DA, Katz E. Multimodal therapy for chronic prostatitis/chronic pelvic pain syndrome. Curr Urol Rep 2005;6:296–9.
18. Dell JR, Butrick CW. Multimodal therapy for painful bladder syndrome/interstitial cystitis. J Reprod Med 2006;51:253–60.
19. Magri V, Wagenlehner F, Perletti G, et al. Use of the UPOINT chronic prostatitis/chronic pelvic pain syndrome classification in European patient cohorts: sexual function domain improves correlations. J Urol 2010;184:2339–45.
20. Shoskes DA, Nickel JC, Dolinga R, et al. Clinical phenotyping of patients with chronic prostatitis/chronic pelvic pain syndrome and correlation with symptom severity. Urology 2009;73:538–42 [discussion: 542–3].
21. Nickel JC, Shoskes D. Phenotypic approach to the management of chronic prostatitis/chronic pelvic pain syndrome. Curr Urol Rep 2009;10:307–12.
22. Nickel JC, Shoskes D, Irvine-Bird K. Clinical phenotyping of women with interstitial cystitis/painful bladder syndrome: a key to classification and potentially improved management. J Urol 2009; 182:155–60.
23. Hedelin HH. Evaluation of a modification of the UPOINT clinical phenotype system for the chronic pelvic pain syndrome. Scand J Urol Nephrol 2009; 43:373–6.
24. Balavoine GG, Geletii YV. Peroxynitrite scavenging by different antioxidants. Part I: convenient assay. Nitric Oxide 1999;3:40–54.

25. Terao J. Dietary flavonoids as antioxidants. Forum Nutr 2009;61:87–94.

26. Chirumbolo S. The role of quercetin, flavonols and flavones in modulating inflammatory cell function. Inflamm Allergy Drug Targets 2010;9:263–85.

27. Bobe G, Albert PS, Sansbury LB, et al. Interleukin-6 as a potential indicator for prevention of high-risk adenoma recurrence by dietary flavonols in the polyp prevention trial. Cancer Prev Res (Phila) 2010;3:764–75.

28. Lee S, Kim YJ, Kwon S, et al. Inhibitory effects of flavonoids on TNF-alpha-induced IL-8 gene expression in HEK 293 cells. BMB Rep 2009;42:265–70.

29. Chuang CC, Martinez K, Xie G, et al. Quercetin is equally or more effective than resveratrol in attenuating tumor necrosis factor-{alpha}-mediated inflammation and insulin resistance in primary human adipocytes. Am J Clin Nutr 2010;92:1511–21.

30. Huang RY, Yu YL, Cheng WC, et al. Immunosuppressive effect of quercetin on dendritic cell activation and function. J Immunol 2010;184:6815–21.

31. He L, Wang Y, Long Z, et al. Clinical significance of IL-2, IL-10, and TNF-alpha in prostatic secretion of patients with chronic prostatitis. Urology 2010;75(3):654–7.

32. Valerio DA, Georgetti SR, Magro DA, et al. Quercetin reduces inflammatory pain: inhibition of oxidative stress and cytokine production. J Nat Prod 2009; 72:1975–9.

33. Hollman PC, Katan MB. Bioavailability and health effects of dietary flavonols in man. Arch Toxicol Suppl 1998;20:237–48.

34. Hertog MG, Feskens EJ, Hollman PC, et al. Dietary antioxidant flavonoids and risk of coronary heart disease: the Zutphen Elderly Study. Lancet 1993;342:1007–11.

35. Kyle JA, Sharp L, Little J, et al. Dietary flavonoid intake and colorectal cancer: a case-control study. Br J Nutr 2010;103:429–36.

36. McCann SE, Ambrosone CB, Moysich KB, et al. Intakes of selected nutrients, foods, and phytochemicals and prostate cancer risk in western New York. Nutr Cancer 2005;53:33–41.

37. Hamdy AA, Ibrahem MA. Management of aphthous ulceration with topical quercetin: a randomized clinical trial. J Contemp Dent Pract 2010;11:E009–16.

38. Egert S, Wolffram S, Bosy-Westphal A, et al. Daily quercetin supplementation dose-dependently increases plasma quercetin concentrations in healthy humans. J Nutr 2008;138:1615–21.

39. Egert S, Bosy-Westphal A, Seiberl J, et al. Quercetin reduces systolic blood pressure and plasma oxidised low-density lipoprotein concentrations in overweight subjects with a high-cardiovascular disease risk phenotype: a double-blinded, placebo-controlled cross-over study. Br J Nutr 2009;102:1065–74.

40. Cruz-Correa M, Shoskes DA, Sanchez P, et al. Combination treatment with curcumin and quercetin of adenomas in familial adenomatous polyposis. Clin Gastroenterol Hepatol 2006;4:1035–8.

41. Shoskes D, Lapierre C, Cruz-Correa M, et al. Beneficial effects of the bioflavonoids curcumin and quercetin on early function in cadaveric renal transplantation: a randomized placebo controlled trial. Transplantation 2005;80:1556–9.

42. Shoskes DA, Zeitlin SI, Shahed A, et al. Quercetin in men with category III chronic prostatitis: a preliminary prospective, double-blind, placebo-controlled trial. Urology 1999;54:960–3.

43. Penna G, Mondaini N, Amuchastegui S, et al. Seminal plasma cytokines and chemokines in prostate inflammation: interleukin 8 as a predictive biomarker in chronic prostatitis/chronic pelvic pain syndrome and benign prostatic hyperplasia. Eur Urol 2007;51:524–33 [discussion: 533].

44. Shahed AR, Shoskes DA. Oxidative stress in prostatic fluid of patients with chronic pelvic pain syndrome: correlation with gram positive bacterial growth and treatment response. J Androl 2000;21: 669–75.

45. Shoskes DA, Albakri Q, Thomas K, et al. Cytokine polymorphisms in men with chronic prostatitis/ chronic pelvic pain syndrome: association with diagnosis and treatment response. J Urol 2002; 168:331–5.

46. Plaper A, Golob M, Hafner I, et al. Characterization of quercetin binding site on DNA gyrase. Biochem Biophys Res Commun 2003;306:530–6.

47. Shoskes DA, Nickel JC, Kattan MW. Phenotypically directed multimodal therapy for chronic prostatitis/ chronic pelvic pain syndrome: a prospective study using UPOINT. Urology 2010;75:1249–53.

48. Pontari MA, McNaughton-Collins M, O'leary MP, et al. A case-control study of risk factors in men with chronic pelvic pain syndrome. BJU Int 2005; 96:559–65.

49. Shoskes D, Prots D, Karns J, et al. Greater endothelial dysfunction and arterial stiffness in men with chronic prostatitis/chronic pelvic pain syndrome- a possible link to cardiovascular disease. J Urol 2011;185(4 Suppl):e572 [abstract: 1428].

Pollen Extract for Chronic Prostatitis— Chronic Pelvic Pain Syndrome

Florian M.E. Wagenlehner, MD, PhD*,
Thomas Bschleipfer, MD, PhD, Adrian Pilatz, MD,
Wolfgang Weidner, MD, PhD

KEYWORDS
- Chronic prostatitis • Chronic pelvic pain syndrome
- Chronic prostatitis symptom index • Pollen extract
- Clinical efficacy

The prostatitis syndrome is mainly characterized by genitourinary pain.[1] Additional symptoms, such as lower urinary tract symptoms, psychosocial symptoms, neurologic symptoms, and sexual dysfunction, might be present in up to 65%.[2] The prevalence of symptoms suggestive of prostatitis in the population ranges between 2.2% and 13.8% according to different studies.[3] The classification of the prostatitis syndrome is best performed by the National Institute of Diabetes and Digestive and Kidney Diseases/National Institutes of Health (NIH)[4] and is classically based on the clinical presentation of a patient, the presence or absence of white blood cells in the expressed prostatic secretion, and the presence or absence of bacteria in the expressed prostatic secretion.[5] Chronic prostatitis–chronic pelvic pain syndrome (CP-CPPS) is the most frequent symptomatic subtype with a heterogenous and mainly unknown etiology. In the NIH classification, bacterial prostatitis (acute and chronic) is distinguished from inflammatory and noninflammatory CP-CPPS.[4] Prostatitis is described as chronic when symptoms are present for at least 3 months. Recently, this classification was clinically amended by a phenotype directed description of patients' symptoms and findings taking into account the various clinical presentations.[2,6]

Etiologically, CP-CPPS may, at least in some patients, be defined by an initial injury to the genitourinary tract (such as infection, trauma, or dysfunctional voiding, in particular in the prostate) causing inflammation and/or neurogenic damage to the prostate, the muscles, fasciae, tendons, and/or nerves of the pelvis and/or perineum in anatomically or genetically predisposed men. This series of events may eventually result in both peripheral and central nervous system sensitization, with pain the common endpoint.[7,8]

Evidence-based treatment of CP-CPPS has been difficult due to the heterogenous patient population associated with this syndrome. Although singular studies provide conflicting results, as in studies of α-blocker therapy,[3,9] meta-analysis data show measurable effects for α-blocker and antiinflammatory therapies.[10] Publication biases in those studies are often due to the common inclusion and exclusion criteria, which frequently did not stratify into phenotypic characteristics that might be targets for the studied agents. Modern therapeutic approaches incorporate considerations of the phenotypic patterns mirroring the possible cause.

Phytotherapeutic agents, such as pollen extract, quercetin, or saw palmetto, are widely used with variable success described in qualitatively heterogenous

Clinic for Urology, Pediatric Urology and Andrology, University Hospital Giessen and Marburg GmbH, Justus Liebig University, Rudolf-Buchheim-Strasse 7, D-35385 Giessen, Germany
* Corresponding author.
E-mail address: Wagenlehner@AOL.com

Urol Clin N Am 38 (2011) 285–292
doi:10.1016/j.ucl.2011.04.004

urologic.theclinics.com

studies.[11–13] The best evidence is currently available for pollen extract. Pollen extract, an herbal medicinal product, has been used for more than 40 years in the treatment of CP-CPPS as well as for benign prostatic hyperplasia.[11,14,15] Pollen extract preparations are merchandised under several product names (Cernilton, Prostat/Poltit, and Pollstimol). Most preclinical studies have been conducted under the preparation name, Cernilton. Data from these studies are discussed in this article. Pollen extract is produced from machine-harvested pollen material from the species, Secale cereale L., Phleum pratense L., and Zea mays L. The proportions of mixture of the 3 species have been constant—30:1.5:1.

Pollen extract is a mixture of natural components, such as amino acids, carbohydrates, lipids, vitamins, and minerals. Phytosterols and secalosides are also believed important constituents in the extract. This highly complex total extract comprises 63 mg of the defined pollen extract fractions constituting 2 main components, the hydrophilic Cernitin T60 fraction and the hydrophobic Cernitin GBX fraction, both of which are devoid of allergenic properties. Inactive ingredients of pollen extract preparations are microcrystalline cellulose, silica, and magnesium stearate.

PHARMACOLOGY

The pharmacology of the total pollen extract and of the 2 pollen extract fractions, Cernitin T60 and Cernitin GBX, primarily, has been studied in different animal models using various modes of administration (oral, gastric intubation, and intraduodenal) and in different species, including mice, rats, and dogs, as well as isolated tissues and cells from different species. These studies revealed spasmogenic and/or spasmolytic effects, antiinflammatory effects, and antiproliferative effects of Cernitin T60 and Cernitin GBX.

Pharmacodynamics

Effects on smooth muscles

At concentrations of 10^{-4} g/mL and higher, Cernitin GBX slightly enhanced the spontaneous movements in the smooth muscles of the intestine and uterus. A spastic action was not observed. In contrast, spasmogenic effects were observed with Cernitin T60. At a concentration of 10^{-5} g/mL, Cernitin T60 led to a slight increase in spasms in the intestine and uterus, whereas at concentrations of 10^{-4} g/mL and higher, there was a definite spastic action.[16]

A synergistic inhibitory effect of Cernitin T60 and Cernitin GBX on noradrenaline-induced contraction of isolated rat urethral muscle was shown by Nakase and colleagues[17] It has been suggested that Cernitin T60 acts on the α-adrenergic receptors whereas Cernitin GBX relaxes the external sphincter and Cernitin extract may relax both the internal and external sphincter muscle.[17]

The total pollen extract contracted isolated detrusor muscles of rats, guinea pigs, and cats in a concentration-dependent manner. Increase of intravesical pressure was reduced completely by atropine and partly by phentolamine and guanethidine. This suggested that Cernitin total extract contracted the detrusor muscle via muscarinic receptor activation causing an increase of the intravesical pressure.[18] Consecutive administration of Cernitin total extract increased the maximum pressure during urination to promote the urination reflex.[19]

The clinical importance of these findings is uncertain, however, because the effects have been observed at relatively high concentrations in vitro.

Antiinflammatory effects

The inhibition of prostaglandin and leukotriene synthesis of pollen extracts has been studied in vitro. Cernitin T60 and Cernitin GBX were tested separately. The inhibition of 5-lipoxygenase activity (leukotriene biosynthesis) by Cernitin GBX was comparable to that of diclofenac and indomethacin, whereas the inhibition of the cyclooxygenase (prostaglandin biosynthesis) was comparable to that of diclofenac and approximately 10 times higher than that of aspirin. Cernitin T60 showed no effect in the test system used.[20]

In an estradiol-17β –induced rat model of nonbacterial prostatitis, an approximately 2-fold to 3-fold increase of prostatic interleukin 6 and tumor necrosis factor α content and an acinar glandular inflammation and stromal proliferation were found in histologic examinations when compared with those of control rats. Pollen extract significantly decreased the increased interleukin 6 and tumor necrosis factor α values in a dose-dependent manner. The histopathologic changes were restored in rats treated with pollen extract as well as in rats treated with testosterone. These findings indicated that pollen extract might have an antiinflammatory effect within the prostate due to an inhibitory effect on the prostatic cytokine content.[21] Further studies have shown that it is mainly Cernitin GBX, which protects the acinar epithelial cells, whereas Cernitin T60 inhibits stromal cell proliferation in association with enhanced apoptosis.[22] In general, the antiinflammatory effect is most likely due to the inhibition of prostaglandin synthesis and prostatic cytokine content related mainly to the Cernitin GBX fraction, which has been shown to have about the same potency as established antiinflammatory agents, such as indomethacine and diclofenac in vitro.

Antiproliferative effects

Varying concentrations of Cernitin GBX were found to inhibit 5α-reductase activity in the epithelium and stroma of the prostate in vitro, inhibiting the formation of dihydrotestosterone from testosterone.[23] Animal studies also found a possible effect on the prostate via the androgen metabolism.[24]

Cernitin T60, furthermore, is a powerful mitogenic inhibitor of fibroblastic and epithelial proliferation. Although the exact mechanism is not understood, not only is there evidence that these responses are mediated via the androgenic pathways[25] but also experimental data in nonbacterial prostatitis in rats showed that Cernitin GBX protects mainly acinar epithelial cells and inhibits stromal proliferation in association with an enhanced apoptosis mediated by Cernitin T-60.[26] The cellular and molecular biology research on growth factors and receptor action indicates that Cernitin T60 and Cernitin GBX affect prostate growth, both with and without growth stimulation.

Pharmacokinetics

Pharmacokinetic studies on the absorption, distribution, metabolism, or excretion of the water-soluble fraction Cernitin T-60 or the lipid-soluble fraction Cernitin GBX have not been performed because it is not known which compounds are primarily responsible for clinical efficacy.

CLINICAL STUDIES

In a cohort of 583 men with chronic prostatitis symptoms or benign prostatic hyperplasia accompanied by chronic prostatitis findings (eg, leukocytes in expressed prostatic secretions higher than 10 per high power field), the number of leukocytes was evaluated before and after a 12-week treatment with pollen extract (Cernilton). The number of leukocytes in expressed prostatic secretions improved to 59% in those patients.[27] These initial findings on the antiinflammatory action of pollen extract led to further evaluate pollen extract in clinical studies investigating its effect on the symptoms of CP-CPPS patients.

Eight clinical studies since then have been performed in patients with CP-CPPS to evaluate the effect of pollen extract on symptoms. Two studies were performed in a randomized placebo-controlled design in 139[13] patients and 58[28] patients. In 6 noncomparative clinical studies, 90, 15, 24, 32, 25, and 106 patients with CP-CPPS were treated.[11,15,29–32] Altogether 392 patients were treated in available studies with pollen extract preparations (Table 1).

Randomized Placebo-Controlled Studies

The largest study, by Wagenlehner and colleagues,[13] was a clinical phase 3 study in 34 German urological centers in 139 patients. Considering the predominantly antiinflammatory effect of pollen extract, this study was performed exclusively in patients with inflammatory CP-CPPS defined by the presence of 10 or more leukocytes in the voided bladder 3 (or post–prostatic massage urine). Patients were randomized to pollen extract or placebo for 12 weeks. In a subsequent open follow-up period of another 12 weeks, all patients received pollen extract. Patients were evaluated by Meares-Stamey 4-glass test and the NIH Chronic Prostatitis Symptom Index (NIH-CPSI)[33] at baseline and after 12 and 24 weeks. Before starting study drugs, patients were pretreated with azithromycin for 1 day to eliminate atypical pathogens. After 1 week, inclusion criteria were rechecked, and patients were included in the treatment phase when both conditions, a pain domain of the NIH-CPSI greater than or equal to 7 and leukocytes greater than or equal to 10 in post–prostatic massage urine, were fulfilled. Patients were then allocated to receive either pollen extract or placebo in a randomized order.

The primary target of the study was symptomatic improvement in the pain domain of the NIH-CPSI. Secondary outcomes included symptomatic improvement of the NIH-CPSI total score and the micturition and quality of life domains of the NIH-CPSI questionnaire, responder assessment defined by improvement of NIH-CPSI summary score by greater than or equal to 25%, or improvement of NIH-CPSI summary score by at least 6 points as well as a decrease in the number of leukocytes in post–prostatic massage urine. Further explorative outcome criteria were changes in the *International Prostate Symptom Score*, the sexuality domain of a life satisfaction questionnaire, residual urine volume, and safety of the study drug. Only results of the intention-to-treat analysis are shown. After 12 weeks of treatment, the mean changes (±SE) from baseline in the pain domain of the NIH-CPSI were −4.50 ± 0.42 in the pollen extract group and −2.92 ± 0.42 in the placebo group ($P = .0086$). The mean NIH-CPSI total score decreased form 19.18 to 11.72 in the pollen extract and from 20.31 to 14.94 in the placebo group ($P = .0126$). Responder analysis showed a significantly greater percentage of patients in the pollen extract group who demonstrated 25% improvement or a 6-point decrease from baseline in the total score compared with

Table 1
Studies performed in patients with CP-CPPS using pollen extract preparations

Product Name	Study Type	Dosage	Duration	Patients (n) in Study	Patients (n) Treated with Pollen Extract	Clinical Response[a]	Refs.
Cernilton	Randomized controlled trial	2 tid	12 (24) Weeks[b]	139	70	69% Pollen extract versus 49% placebo (P = .015) >25% Improvement NIH-CPSI or 6-point decrease of NIH-CPSI[a]	13,34
Prostat/Poltit	Randomized controlled trial	NI	6 Months	58	30	73% Pollen extract versus 36% placebo (P<.05) Global subjective assessment[a]	28
Cernilton N	Cohort study	1 tid	6 Months	90	90	63% Global objective assessment[a]	11
Cernilton	Cohort study	2 bid	1 to 8 Months	15	15	87% Global subjective assessment[a]	15
Cernilton	Cohort study	3 tid	4 to 6 Weeks	24	24	63% >50% improvement NIH-CPSI[a]	29
Cernilton	Cohort study	2 tid	12 Weeks	32	32	66% Global objective assessment[a]	31
Cernilton	Cohort study	2 tid	8 Weeks	25	25	76% Global objective assessment[a]	32
Prostat/Poltit	Cohort study	NI	8 Weeks	106	106	NI	30

Abbreviation: NI, not indicated in publication.
[a] Responder criteria not uniform.
[b] Trial extension period 24 weeks, with all patients receiving pollen extract from week 12 on.

the placebo group (P = .0147 and P = .0256, respectively). The mean quality-of-life domain of the NIH-CPSI decreased from 6.44 to 4.26 in the pollen extract group and from 6.68 to 5.28 in the placebo group (P = .0250). The mean changes from baseline in the number of leukocytes per field of vision were 5.0 in the pollen extract group and 3.0 in the placebo group (P = .1243). The global assessment of the efficacy by the patient showed significantly higher rates of very good or good results in the pollen extract group (62.9%) compared with the placebo group (41.8%).

A total of 93 patients completed the follow-up period up to 24 weeks in which patients in the placebo arm crossed over to receive pollen extract. Thus 48 patients from the pollen extract arm continued to receive pollen extract up to week 24, and 45 patients in the placebo arm received pollen extract from weeks 12 to 24.[34] The pain, quality-of-life domains, and the total NIH-CPSI score continued to improve at week 24 in both groups. The latter effects were more pronounced in patients with crossover from placebo to pollen extract from week 12 on. Urinary symptoms improved moderately, but not significantly, in both groups. Leukocytes in the post-prostatic massage urine improved significantly in both groups at week 12 and continued to improve at week 24 in both groups, with a more pronounced effect in the initial pollen extract arm. Adverse events were minor in all patients.

The conclusion of this study was that pollen extract compared with placebo significantly improved total symptoms, pain, and quality-of-life and reduced leukocytes in the post–massage urine in patients with inflammatory CP-CPPS without severe side effects up to 24 weeks. The beneficial effect continued to improve after 12 weeks' treatment showing that pollen extract can be recommended for patients with inflammatory CP-CPPS for long-term treatment.

Randomized placebo-controlled study in patients with inflammatory or noninflammatory CP-CPPS

In a monocenter study by Elist, 58 patients with inflammatory or noninflammatory CP-CPPS were included.[28] For inclusion in this study, no cutoff NIH-CPSI value was reported; case number calculations were also not reported. Patients were randomized to pollen extract or placebo for 6 months. Primary or secondary outcome variables were not discussed in the publication, but the analysis included data on pain and lower urinary tract symptoms, evaluated by a modified University of Washington symptom score, sexual dysfunction and an overall clinical response at

baseline and after 24 weeks. Mean changes ($\pm$SE) from baseline in the pain symptom domain of the modified University of Washington symptom score were -6.70 ± 4.5 in the pollen extract group and -1.7 ± 3.2 in the placebo group, which were described as significant. Lower urinary tract symptoms also were reduced to a higher extent in the pollen extract arm compared with the placebo arm; sexual function was better in the pollen extract arm after 6 months' treatment. The overall clinical response showed that 73% of patients were considered clinically improved or cured in the pollen extract arm, whereas in the placebo group only 36% of patients were considered improved. The investigators concluded that pollen extract administered for 6 months would ameliorate the symptoms associated with CP-CPPS effectively.[28]

Nonrandomized studies in patients with CP-CPPS

In a study by Rugendorff and colleagues,[11] 90 patients were prospectively treated with pollen extract (1 tablet 3 times a day for 6 months). Patients were assessed before and after 3 and 6 months' treatment by physical examination, bacterial studies, leukocyte counts in urine, and measurement of complement C3/coeruloplasmin in the seminal fluid. For further analysis, the patients were divided into 2 groups: those without associated complicating factors (CFs) (n = 72) and those with CFs (ie, urethral strictures, prostatic calculi, and bladder neck sclerosis [n = 18]). In the group without CFs, 78% had a favorable response, 36% were cured, and 42% improved significantly. In the patients with CFs, only 1 patient showed a response. The investigators concluded that CFs should be considered in patients who fail to respond to treatment within 3 months.

In another open study by Buck and colleagues,[15] 15 patients with CP-CPPS were treated with pollen extract (2 tablets twice a day for 1 to 18 months). In 13 patients there was either complete and lasting relief of symptoms or a marked improvement; 2 patients failed to respond. The investigators concluded that pollen extract was found effective in 87% of patients with CP-CPPS.

In a study by Monden and colleagues,[29] 24 patients with CP-CPPS (16 patients with inflammatory CP-CPPS and 8 with noninflammatory CP-CPPS) were treated with pollen extract. Examination of changes in the NIH-CPSI scores revealed that scores of the items in all domains were significantly lower 4 to 6 weeks after the start of administration of Cernilton than those obtained before the drug administration in patients with CP-CPPS. In 62.5% of cases, the total NIH-CPSI score improved more than 50% compared with baseline. There was no difference between inflammatory and noninflammatory CP-CPPS patients.

A study by Li and colleagues[30] was performed in 106 patients with CP-CPPS treated with pollen extract for 8 weeks and the mean NIH-CPSI score was significantly reduced from 24.1 at baseline to 12.2 at the end of treatment.

A study by Jodai and colleagues[31] was another open study in 32 patients who received pollen extract for 12.6 weeks on the average. Improvement of subjective symptoms and objective findings was observed in 74.2% and 65.6% of the cases, respectively. The effective rate was reported to be 75.0%. No subjective symptoms or abnormal changes in laboratory data were observed in any case after pollen extract medication.[31]

Another study was performed by Suzuki and colleagues[32] in 25 patients with CP-CPPS treated with pollen extract for 8 weeks and longer. There was improvement of subjective symptoms and objective findings in 96.0% and 76.0%, respectively, of the cases. No side effects were observed.[32]

In all studies, pollen extract was tolerated well by the patients over the extended periods of time.

DISCUSSION

Although in chronic bacterial prostatitis, antibiotic treatment is the standard,[35] there is no standard treatment of CP-CPPS up to date.[36,37] Although many studies in different qualities have been performed, current trial evidence is conflicting and therapeutic options are controversial. A variety of treatment options are reported, such as α-blocker therapies,[3,9] antibiotics, antiinflammatory agents, phytotherapeutics, and various other treatments.[11,15,38–43] All treatment modalities, however, showed heterogenous and limited effects on the symptoms experienced in CP-CPPS, of which pain and dysfunctional voiding cause the greatest morbidity and a poor quality of life.[44] Not all of the studies have been performed in adequate randomized placebo-controlled design. In a systematic review and network meta-analysis, α-blockers, antibiotics, and combinations of these therapies seemed to achieve the greatest improvement in clinical symptom scores, if compared with placebo, although the beneficial effects of α-blockers may have been overestimated because of publication bias.[10] Antiinflammatory therapies had a lesser but measurable benefit on selected outcomes.[10] Studies of antiinflammatory action have mainly been performed in patients without necessarily the evidence of inflammation. Therefore, a better

selection of patients for study inclusion might lead to improved outcome as shown in the phenotypical approach.[45] Signs of inflammation within the prostate or other prostate-specific factors, for example, are frequently found in up to 84% of CP-CPPS patients.[2]

Given the lack of proved efficacy of conventional therapies and the need for long-term treatment in CP-CPPS patients, alternative treatment options are urgently needed. Phytotherapeutics are, therefore, an option, due to their generally few side effects, but few substances have been subjected to scientific scrutiny and prospective controlled clinical trials, among which are pollen extract, quercetin, saw palmetto, and terpenes.[15,39–41]

Pollen extract has been evaluated sufficiently in preclinical and clinical studies. Pharmacodynamic investigations have shown effects on smooth muscles of the bladder and urethra, strong antiinflammatory effects, and antiproliferative effects.[16–26]

Two pollen extract preparations have been assessed in various clinical studies under the names, Cernilton and Prostat/Poltit. Six clinical studies have been performed with Cernilton (1 randomized controlled trial and 5 cohort studies) in 256 patients receiving the active substance and 2 clinical studies have been performed with Prostat/Poltit (2 randomized controlled trial and 1 cohort study) in 136 patients (see **Table 1**). Clinical efficacy was evaluated heterogeneously in the different studies but ranged between 63% and 87%. In the 2 placebo-controlled studies, the clinical response was significantly better in the pollen extract groups compared with the placebo groups, although efficacy rates in the placebo groups reached 36% and 49% (see **Table 1**).

In all the studies, both pollen extract preparations were generally well tolerated over the full study periods.

SUMMARY

Pollen extract preparations have been investigated sufficiently in preclinical and clinical studies in patients with CP-CPPS. Pharmacodynamic investigations of pollen extract have shown relaxing effects on internal and external sphincter smooth muscles of the bladder and urethra, strong antiinflammatory effects, and antiproliferative effects. Clinical studies revealed improvement or cure of symptoms in 63% to 87% of patients with CP-CPPS, significantly superior to placebo in the randomized controlled studies. Long-term treatment is necessary and in all the studies pollen extract preparations were generally well tolerated over the full study periods.

REFERENCES

1. Schaeffer AJ. Clinical practice. Chronic prostatitis and the chronic pelvic pain syndrome. N Engl J Med 2006;355(16):1690–8.

2. Magri V, Wagenlehner F, Perletti G, et al. Use of the UPOINT chronic prostatitis/chronic pelvic pain syndrome classification in European patient cohorts: sexual function domain improves correlations. J Urol 2010;184(6):2339–45.

3. Schaeffer AJ, Anderson, RU, Krieger, JN, et al. The assessment and management of male pelvic pain syndrome, including prostatitis. Committee 15. In: McConnell J, Abrams P, Denis L, et al, editors. Male Lower Urinary tract dysfunction. Evaluation and Management. 9th International Consultation on New Developments in Prostate Cancer and Prostatitic Diseases, Paris (France), June 24–27, 2005; Health Publications: 2006. p. 341–75.

4. Krieger JN, Nyberg L Jr, Nickel JC. NIH consensus definition and classification of prostatitis. JAMA 1999;282(3):236–7.

5. Schaeffer AJ. Prostatitis: US perspective. Int J Antimicrob Agents 1999;11(3–4):205–11 [discussion: 213–6].

6. Shoskes DA, Nickel JC, Dolinga R, et al. Clinical phenotyping of patients with chronic prostatitis/chronic pelvic pain syndrome and correlation with symptom severity. Urology 2009;73(3):538–42 [discussion: 542–3].

7. Gonzalez RR, Te AE. Chronic prostatitis and sensory urgency: whose pain is it? Curr Urol Rep 2004;5(6): 437–41.

8. Karlovsky ME, Pontari MA. Theories of prostatitis etiology. Curr Urol Rep 2002;3(4):307–12.

9. Nickel JC, Krieger JN, McNaughton-Collins M, et al. Alfuzosin and symptoms of chronic prostatitis-chronic pelvic pain syndrome. N Engl J Med 2008; 359(25):2663–73.

10. Anothaisintawee T, Attia J, Nickel JC, et al. Management of chronic prostatitis/chronic pelvic pain syndrome: a systematic review and network meta-analysis. JAMA 2011;305(1):78–86.

11. Rugendorff EW, Weidner W, Ebeling L, et al. Results of treatment with pollen extract (Cernilton N) in chronic prostatitis and prostatodynia. Br J Urol 1993;71(4):433–8.

12. Shoskes DA. Phytotherapy in chronic prostatitis. Urology 2002;60(Suppl 6):35–7 [discussion: 37].

13. Wagenlehner FM, Schneider H, Ludwig M, et al. A pollen extract (Cernilton) in patients with inflammatory chronic prostatitis-chronic pelvic pain syndrome: a multicentre, randomised, prospective, double-blind, placebo-controlled phase 3 study. Eur Urol 2009;56(3):544–51.

14. Buck AC, Cox R, Rees RW, et al. Treatment of outflow tract obstruction due to benign prostatic hyperplasia with the pollen extract, cernilton. A double-blind, placebo-controlled study. Br J Urol 1990;66(4):398–404.

15. Buck AC, Rees RW, Ebeling L. Treatment of chronic prostatitis and prostatodynia with pollen extract. Br J Urol 1989;64(5):496–9.

16. Pharmacological Studies of CERNILTON, Cernitin GBX and Cernitin T60. Tokyo: Tobishi Pharmaceutical Co., LTD; 1968.

17. Nakase K, Takenag K, Hamanaka T, et al. Inhibitory effect and synergism of Cernitin extract on the urethral smooth muscle and diaphragm of the rat. Nippon Yakurigaku Zasshi 1988;91:385–92 [in Japanese].

18. Onodera S, Yoshinaga M, Takenaga K, et al. Effects of Cernitin extract (CN-009) on the isolated bladder smooth muscles and the intravesical pressure. Nippon Yakurigaku Zasshi 1991;97:267–76.

19. Nagashima A, Ishii M, Yoshinaga M, et al. Effect of Cernitin extract (Cernilton) on the function of urinary bladder in conscious rats. Japan Pharmacol Ther 1998;26(11).

20. Loschen G, Ebeling L. Inhibition of arachidonic acid cascade by extract of rye pollen. Arzneimittelforschung 1991;41(2):162–7 [in German].

21. Asakawa K, Nandachi N, Satoh S, et al. Effects of cernitin pollen-extract (Cernilton) on inflammatory cytokines in sex-hormone-induced nonbacterial prostatitis rats. Hinyokika Kiyo 2001;47(7):459–65.

22. Kawakami J, Siemens DR, Nickel JC. Prostatitis and prostate cancer: implications for prostate cancer screening. Urology 2004;64(6):1075–80.

23. Tunn S, Krieg M. Alterations in the intraprostatic hormonal metabolism by the pollen extract Cernilton. In: Vahlensieck W, Rutischauser G, editors. Benign prostate diseases. Stuttgart (Germany); New York: Georg Thieme Verlag; 1992. p. 109–14.

24. Talpur N, Echard B, Bagchi D, et al. Comparison of Saw Palmetto (extract and whole berry) and Cernitin on prostate growth in rats. Mol Cell Biochem 2003; 250(1–2):21–6.

25. Habib FK. Regulation of prostate growth in culture with the Pollen Extract Cernitin T60 and the impact of the drug on the EGF tissue profile. In: Vahlensieck W, Rutishauser G, editors. Benign prostate diseases. Stuttgart (Germany); New York: Georg Thieme Verlag; 1992. p. 115–22.

26. Kamijo T, Sato S, Kitamura T. Effect of cernitin pollen-extract on experimental nonbacterial prostatitis in rats. Prostate 2001;49(2):122–31.

27. Ebeling L. Therapeutic results of defined Pollen-extract in patients with chronic prostatitis or BPH accompanied by chronic prostatitis. In: Weidner W, Brunner H, Krause W, et al, editors. Therapy of prostatitis. München (Germany); Bern, Wien, San Francisco: Zuckerschwerd; 1986. p. 154–60.

28. Elist J. Effects of pollen extract preparation Prostat/Poltit on lower urinary tract symptoms in patients

with chronic nonbacterial prostatitis/chronic pelvic pain syndrome: a randomized, double-blind, placebo-controlled study. Urology 2006;67(1):60–3.

29. Monden K, Tsugawa M, Ninomiya Y, et al. A Japanese version of the National Institutes of Health Chronic Prostatitis Symptom Index (NIH-CPSI, Okayama version) and the clinical evaluation of cernitin pollen extract for chronic non-bacterial prostatitis. Nippon Hinyokika Gakkai Zasshi 2002;93(4):539–47 [in Japanese].

30. Li NC, Na YQ, Guo HQ. Clinical study with Prostat (Poltit) for treatment for chronic nonbacterial prostatitis. Chin J Urol 2003;24:635–7.

31. Jodai A, Maruta N, Shimomae E, et al. A long-term therapeutic experience with Cernilton in chronic prostatitis. Hinyokika Kiyo 1988;34(3):561–8 [in Japanese].

32. Suzuki T, Kurokawa K, Mashimo T, et al. Clinical effect of Cernilton in chronic prostatitis. Hinyokika Kiyo 1992;38(4):489–94 [in Japanese].

33. Hochreiter W, Ludwig M, Weidner W, et al. National Institutes of Health (NIH) Chronic Prostatitis Symptom Index. The German version. Urologe A 2001;40(1):16–7 [in German].

34. Wagenlehner FME, Schneider H, Ludwig M, et al. Long term efficacy of Cernilton in patients with chronic prostatitis/chronic pelvic pain syndrome type NIH IIIA [abstract 559]. Eur Urol Suppl 2009;8(4):260.

35. Bjerklund Johansen TE, Gruneberg RN, Guibert J, et al. The role of antibiotics in the treatment of chronic prostatitis: a consensus statement. Eur Urol 1998;34(6):457–66.

36. Tugcu V, Tasci AI, Fazlioglu A, et al. A placebo-controlled comparison of the efficiency of triple- and monotherapy in category III B chronic pelvic pain syndrome (CPPS). Eur Urol 2007;51(4):1113–7 [discussion: 1118].

37. Naber KG, Bergman B, Bishop MC, et al. EAU guidelines for the management of urinary and male genital tract infections. Urinary Tract Infection (UTI) Working Group of the Health Care Office (HCO) of the European Association of Urology (EAU). Eur Urol 2001;40(5):576–88.

38. Capodice JL, Bemis DL, Buttyan R, et al. Complementary and alternative medicine for chronic prostatitis/chronic pelvic pain syndrome. Evid Based Complement Alternat Med 2005;2(4):495–501.

39. Lee CB, Ha US, Lee SJ, et al. Preliminary experience with a terpene mixture versus ibuprofen for treatment of category III chronic prostatitis/chronic pelvic pain syndrome. World J Urol 2006;24(1):55–60.

40. Kaplan SA, Volpe MA, Te AE. A prospective, 1-year trial using saw palmetto versus finasteride in the treatment of category III prostatitis/chronic pelvic pain syndrome. J Urol 2004;171(1):284–8.

41. Shoskes DA, Zeitlin SI, Shahed A, et al. Quercetin in men with category III chronic prostatitis: a preliminary prospective, double-blind, placebo-controlled trial. Urology 1999;54(6):960–3.

42. Shoskes DA. Phytotherapy and other alternative forms of care for the patient with prostatitis. Curr Urol Rep 2002;3(4):330–4.

43. Nickel JC, Pontari M, Moon T, et al. A randomized, placebo controlled, multicenter study to evaluate the safety and efficacy of rofecoxib in the treatment of chronic nonbacterial prostatitis. J Urol 2003;169(4):1401–5.

44. Nickel JC. Role of alpha1-blockers in chronic prostatitis syndromes. BJU Int 2008;101(Suppl 3):11–6.

45. Shoskes DA, Nickel JC, Kattan MW. Phenotypically directed multimodal therapy for chronic prostatitis/chronic pelvic pain syndrome: a prospective study using UPOINT. Urology 2010;75(6):1249–53.

Lifestyle/Dietary Recommendations for Erectile Dysfunction and Female Sexual Dysfunction

Katherine Esposito, MD, PhD[a],*, Dario Giugliano, MD, PhD[b]

KEYWORDS

- Lifestyle changes • Recommendations
- Erectile dysfunction • Female sexual dysfunction

Erectile dysfunction (ED) is defined as the consistent inability to attain or maintain a penile erection of sufficient quality to permit satisfactory sexual intercourse. ED is an important cause of decreased quality of life in men.[1] It has been estimated that the worldwide prevalence of ED will be 322 million cases by the year 2025.[2] The prevalence of this condition increases with age,[3] although ED cannot be defined as necessary consequence of aging. There has been increasing recognition of the many physiologic causes of ED and of the potential for therapy to improve a patient's quality of life, self-esteem, and ability to maintain intimate relationships.[4] Although epidemiologic evidence seems to support a role for lifestyle factors, limited data are available suggesting that the treatment of underlying risk factors and coexisting illnesses—for example with diet, exercise, and smoking cessation—may improve ED.[5]

The definition of female sexual dysfunction (FSD) includes persistent or recurrent disorders of sexual interest/desire, disorders of subjective and genital arousal, orgasmic disorders, pain, and difficulty with attempted or incomplete intercourse.[6] The debate as to whether FSD should be classified as a dysfunction similar to ED or whether it should be considered a pathologic condition at all is not ended. A study of a US population[1] showed that women reported sexual dysfunction more often than men (43% vs 31%), and 20% women were seeking medical consultation for sexual dysfunction. Moreover, approximately 22% of these women reported feeling distressed by their sexual dysfunction.[7] These percentages have recently been confirmed by the results of Global Study of Sexual Attitudes and Behaviors, an international survey of various aspects of gender and relationships among adults aged 40 to 80 years.[8] Well-designed, random sample, community-based epidemiologic studies, however, are limited and hampered by low response rate, the use of different tools to assess FSD, and the underlying complexity of female sexuality.

LIFESTYLE FACTORS AND SEXUAL FUNCTION

Healthy behaviors are associated with a reduced risk for ED. In the Health Professionals Follow-Up Study,[9] for example, several modifiable lifestyle factors, including normal weight, increased physical activity, nonsmoking, moderate alcohol consumption, and less television viewing, were associated with maintenance of good erectile function. The results are sparse regarding

The authors have nothing to disclose.

[a] Department of Cardio-Thoracic and Respiratory Sciences, Second University of Naples, Piazza L. Miraglia 2, 80138 Naples, Italy

[b] Department of Geriatrics and Metabolic Diseases, Second University of Naples, Piazza L. Miraglia 2, 80138 Naples, Italy

* Corresponding author.

E-mail address: katherine.esposito@unina2.it

doi:10.1016/j.ucl.2011.04.006
0094-0143/11/$ – see front matter

urologic.theclinics.com

associations between lifestyle factors and FSD, and conclusions regarding potential influence of healthy behaviors on FSD cannot be made before more studies have been performed.

Overweight and Obesity

Both cross-sectional and prospective epidemiologic studies suggest that overweight and obesity are associated with an increased risk of ED.[10] In particular, the largest population from the Health Professionals Follow-Up Study in the United States, including 31,724 men free of ED at baseline, showed a 40% increased risk of developing ED with obesity.[9] Prospective studies[11–13] of variable duration from 5 to 25 years of follow-up reported that overweight or obese men had an increased probability (70% to 96% higher) of developing ED compared with normal weight men.

Few studies have investigated the association between obesity and female sexual satisfaction, with nonunivocal results. In a Swedish population studied by Adolfsson and colleagues[14] of 840 younger women (18–49 years) and 426 older women (50–74 years), there was no difference in satisfaction of sexual life between obese and normal weight women, although there was a tendency toward lower sexual satisfaction and sexual desire associated with higher weights in the youngest age group. In 1158 women and men, who were participating in an intensive residential program for weight loss and lifestyle modification or were evaluated for gastric bypass surgery or were obese control subjects not seeking weight loss treatment, approximately 50% of obese women (54.7% to 61.2%) reported difficulty with these aspects of sexual quality of life at least some of the time.[15] The authors and colleagues found[16] a strong negative relationship (r = −0.72) between body weight and sexual function in 52 women with abnormal values of the Female Sexual Function Index (FSFI).

Physical Activity

There is evidence for a protective effect of increased physical activity on ED. In the Health Professionals Follow-Up Study,[9] men in the highest quintile of physical activity were likely to carry a 30% lower risk for ED than those in the referent quintile (sedentary men); in addition, watching television for more than 20 hours per week was also significantly associated with ED (relative risk 1.2) after controlling for leisure physical activity and other health-related factors. A recent meta-analysis of population-based studies demonstrates the existence of a simple dose-response relationship, with higher physical activity conferring

lower risks: the adjusted reduction of the risk of having ED was 58% for high activity and 37% for moderate activity compared with men with low physical activity.[17] In a more recent study of 674 men aged 45 to 60 years examined at their place of work,[18] the risk of severe ED was decreased by 82.9% for men with physical activity of at least 3000 kcal per week compared with men under 3000 kcal per week (P = .018).

There are few studies available that specifically investigated the association between physical activity and FSD. The Boston Area Community Health (BACH) survey was a 2002–2005 community-based epidemiologic study of urologic and gynecologic symptoms, sociodemographics, health status, and psychosocial characteristics in a diverse sample of Boston area residents (N = 3205 women aged 30–79 years). Analyses of sexual problems and their correlates were conducted for the subset of women who engaged in sexual activity with a partner in the previous 4 weeks.[19] A total of 49% of participants were not sexually active, citing lack of interest (51.5%) and lack of a partner (60.8%) as the most common reasons. The likelihood of sexual activity increased with physical activity (odds ratio 1.84, high vs low physical activity level). In a small series of women evaluated prospectively during the natural traverse of menopause, with questionnaires administered at years 1 and year 5, exercise was the only variable associated with sexual satisfaction.[20] In 458 sexually active women participating in the ongoing 5-year longitudinal study, cross-sectional analysis of sexual functioning data revealed that irrespective of stage of menopause, being physically active (at least 30 minutes of physical activity 5 days a week) was associated with higher level of engagement and enjoyment.[21] In 595 women with type 2 diabetes mellitus who completed the FSFI questionnaire, those with higher levels of physical activity were approximately 10% less likely to have FSD compared with those with the lowest level of physical activity.[22]

Smoking

Smoking seems a consolidated risk factor for ED, because it doubles the risk, and passive (secondhand) smoking also increases the risk of ED.[11] Smoking was also correlated with increased ED in the Health Professionals Follow-Up Study, with a 30% increased risk of ED in current smokers compared with nonsmokers.[9] These results have been refined by the publication of a more recent assessment of this population, with a 14-year follow-up period and 3905 new cases of ED from 22,086 participants[23]: smoking was a positive risk factor for ED, both for past smokers (relative risk of 1.1) and current smokers (relative risk 1.4).

There are few studies exploring the relation between smoking and female sexual function. In the Women's Health Initiative observational study,[24] sexual satisfaction was not associated with smoking in 46,525 respondents answering the sexual satisfaction question. In the BACH survey, smoking history did not modify the probability of having sexual problems.[19] In 595 women with type 2 diabetes mellitus, no association was found between cigarette smoking status and FSD.[22]

Alcohol

Alcohol intake has been associated with decreased ED,[9] probably in part because of the long-term benefits of alcohol on high-density lipoprotein cholesterol and other variables that increase the bioavailability of nitric oxide. In the BACH survey,[25] a multistage stratified random sample was used to recruit 2301 men ages 30 to 79 years from the city of Boston between 2002 and 2005: the results showed a positive, albeit nonsignificant, association with the International Index of Erectile Function (IIEF) score, which was highest with 1 to 3 drinks per day. The data from a population-based cross-sectional study of men's health to assess the association between usual alcohol consumption and ED in Australia revealed that among current drinkers (n = 1374), the odds were lowest for consumption between 1 and 20 standard drinks per week.[26] On further adjustment for cardiovascular disease (CVD) or for cigarette smoking, age-adjusted odds of ED were reduced by 25% to 30% among alcohol drinkers. In general, the overall findings are suggestive of alcohol consumption of moderate quantity conferring the highest protection.[27]

The studies addressing the relation between alcohol consumption and sexual function in women are scanty. In the 3205 women aged 30 to 79 years participating in the BACH survey,[19] the likelihood of sexual activity increased with alcohol consumption (odds ratio 7.63 ≥3 drinks/day vs none).

Diet and Dietary Habits

Subjects with ED seem to have a vascular mechanism similar to that seen in atherosclerosis[28] and, therefore, a diagnosis of ED may be seen as a sentinel event that should prompt investigation for coronary heart disease (CHD) in asymptomatic men. It seems, therefore, reasonable to assume that dietary factors, which are important in reducing the burden of CHD disease,[29] may also play a role in reducing the occurrence of ED. Physiologic differences in sexual functioning between men and women exist, however, which may relevant to the association between FSD and CHD. In the Women's Health Initiative observational study,[24] 35,719 respondents women reported satisfaction with sexual activity. There was no increased prevalence or incidence of CVD among sexually active female subjects complaining of dissatisfaction with sexual activity at baseline over 7.8 years of follow-up, and dissatisfaction did not predict incident CVD.

As intriguing this hypothesis is, there are few studies that have assessed the link of diet in ED. The intake of some foods may be less represented in subjects with ED. In a case-control study exploring this relation, the authors compared 100 men who had ED without diabetes and CVD, with 100 age-matched and disease-matched men who did not have ED.[30] In analyses adjusted for the prevalence of associated risk factors, the intake of vegetables, fruits, and nuts and the ratio of monounsaturated lipids to saturated lipids remained the only individual measures associated with ED. In 555 men with type 2 diabetes mellitus attending diabetes clinics located in the area of the Campania County, South Italy, the authors assessed the relation between adherence to Mediterranean diet and sexual function.[31] Median intakes of food groups associated with a Mediterranean diet were calculated, and the participants received a point on the scale if they measured above the median consumption for fish, fruit, legumes, nuts, ratio of monounsaturated to saturated fat, vegetables, and whole grains; otherwise, they received 0 points. Red and processed meat consumption below the median received 1 point, otherwise 0 points. For ethanol, a value of 1 was assigned to men who consumed between 10 and 50 g per day and to women who consumed 5 to 25 g per day. Thus, Mediterranean dietary pattern scores ranged from 0 to 9; higher scores indicated closer adherence to a Mediterranean-type diet. The overall prevalence of ED among diabetic men showed a progressive and significant decline across tertiles: men with the highest score of adherence to the Mediterranean diet had the lowest global prevalence of ED, which remained significant in multivariate analysis that included confounding factors.

The relation between consumption of a Mediterranean-type diet and sexual function has been evaluated in a population of 595 women with type 2 diabetes mellitus, aged 35 to 70 years.[32] Based on the FSFI cutoff score for FSD of 23, women with the highest score of adherence had a lower prevalence of sexual dysfunction compared with women of lower tertiles (47.6%, 53.9%, and 57.8% corresponding to higher, middle, and lower tertiles, respectively; $P = .01$) (**Fig. 1**).

Lifestyle Changes and Sexual Function

In general, the validity of the studies can be discussed, because most studies include few participants or short follow-up periods or suffer from selection bias. These studies evaluated the effect of intensive lifestyle changes aimed at reducing body weight and increasing physical activity or investigated the effect of any single component, such as weight loss, increased physical activity, or a particular dietary pattern.

Overall lifestyle changes

Esposito and colleagues[33] looked at the effect of weight loss and increased physical activity on ED in 55 obese men with ED compared with 55 matched-controls, measuring elevated levels of

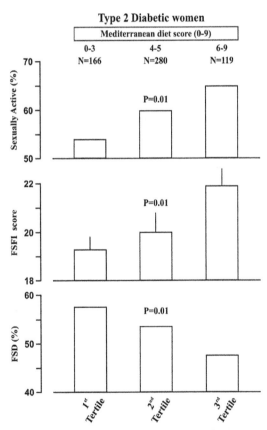

Fig. 1. Relation between adherence to Mediterranean diet and FSD in women with type 2 diabetes mellitus. Adherence to a Mediterranean diet was scored in tertiles, from the lowest (score 0–3 points) to the highest (score 6–9 points) adherence. There was a linear relation between adherence to a Mediterranean diet and the prevalence of FSD.

proinflammatory cytokines as a marker of inflammation and endothelial function, and using these markers as an indication of ED. Men assigned to the intervention group were entered in an intensive weight loss program, involving personalized dietary counseling and exercise advice and regular meetings with a nutritionist and personal trainer. The dietary advice was tailored to each man on the basis of food records collected on 3 nonconsecutive days, which had to be done the week before the meeting with a nutritionist. Men in the control group were given general oral and written information about healthy food choices and exercise at baseline and at subsequent bimonthly visits, but no specific individualized programs were offered to them. After 2 years, men randomized to the intervention had lost significantly more weight, increased their physical activity, experienced favorable changes in physiologic measures of endothelial dysfunction, and had significant improvement in their ED score compared with men in the control group. The investigators suggested that the improvement in ED was a potential effect of the endothelial function following the improvement in the inflammatory markers.

Wing and colleagues[34] examined 1-year changes in erectile function in 306 overweight men with type 2 diabetes mellitus participating in the Look AHEAD (Action for Health in Diabetes) trial: in participants assigned to intensive lifestyle intervention (group or individual sessions to reduce weight and increase physical activity), 8% reported a worsening of EF from baseline to 1 year, whereas the percentage in the control participants was 22%. The overall IIEF score improved from 17.3 to 18.6 in the intervention group.

The authors used their database of subjects participating in randomized controlled trials to see whether improvement of erectile function was related to success in achieving lifestyle changes.[35] A total of 209 subjects were randomly assigned to 1 of the 2 treatment groups. The 104 men randomly assigned to the intervention program received detailed advice about how to reduce body weight, improve quality of diet, and increase physical activity. The goals of the intervention were a reduction in weight of 5% or more, a reduction in intake of saturated fat to less than 10% of energy consumed, an increase in intake of monounsaturated fat to 10% or more of energy consumed, an increase in fiber intake to at least 15 g per 1000 kcal, and moderate exercise for at least 30 minutes per day for at least 5 days in a week. The study subjects were ranked according to their success in achieving the goals of the intervention (and given a success score between 0 and 5) at the 2-year examination, with higher scores indicating more goals met: there was a strong correlation between the success score and restoration of erectile function. At the end, men without ED were significantly higher in the intervention group compared with men in the control group (**Fig. 2**).

Weight loss

Kolotkin and colleagues[36] examined the effect of weight loss on quality of life, including 6 questions about sexual life among 37 men and women, with no information about the intervention or the achieved weight loss from this intervention. After a follow-up of 28 days, the weight loss program seemed to have been beneficial among men, whereas among women there was no association between weight changes and changes in sexual life. Werlinger and colleagues[37] demonstrated that weight loss significantly increased the overall perception of sexual functioning and increased sexual satisfaction in 32 women with an average follow-up of 31 weeks. Kaukua and colleagues[38] measured the effect of weight loss on changes in sex hormones and sexual function among 38 obese men. The men followed a 10-week very-low-energy diet and behavior modification and maintenance of weight loss for 8 months. The study did not show significant treatment effect on sexual functioning. A more recent study by Kolotkin and colleagues[39] evaluated changes in sexual quality of life over a 2-year period in 187 adults (161 women and 26 men) undergoing weight loss treatment. Weight loss averaged

13% and was significantly associated with improvements in sexual quality of life, with women more likely to improve all dimensions of quality of life than men.

Khoo and colleagues[40] compared the effects of 8 weeks of a low-calorie diet using meal replacements (KicStart) on insulin sensitivity; plasma testosterone levels; erectile function (IIEF-5); and sexual desire as measured by the Sexual Desire Inventory in abdominally obese (body mass index >30 and waist >102 cm) men with uncomplicated diabetes (n = 19) or without type 2 diabetes mellitus (n = 25) with a control group of nondiabetic men (n = 26) with similar body mass index and waist circumference. Weight loss of 10% was significantly associated with increased insulin sensitivity, plasma testosterone levels, and IIEF-5 and Sexual Desire Inventory scores in diabetic as well as nondiabetic men.

Physical activity

White and colleagues[41] examined the effect of 9 months' exercise on sexuality among 78 healthy, sedentary men, and showed that sedentary behaviors were associated with ED risk. Specifically, they found that the intervention (60 minutes/day, approximately 3.5 days/week at 75% to 80% maximum aerobic capacity) significantly enhanced the frequency of intercourse, orgasms, and maintained erections as recorded in sexuality diaries of the exercising group compared with the control group who were prescribed a low-intensity walking program.

Dietary pattern

The specific role of diet was assessed by the analysis the effect of Mediterranean diet on ED in subjects with the metabolic syndrome.[42] Sixty-five men with the metabolic syndrome and ED were enrolled in the study; 35 out of them were assigned to the intervention diet and 30 to the control diet. Subjects in the intervention group were advised to consume at least 250 to 300 g of fruits, 125 to 150 g of vegetables, and 25 to 50 g of nuts per day; in addition, they were encouraged to consume 400 g of whole grains daily (legumes, rice, maize, and wheat) and to increase the consumption of olive oil. After 2 years, men on the Mediterranean diet consumed a greater percentage of calories from polyunsaturated and monounsaturated fat; had a greater intake of ω-3 fatty acids; and had lower saturated fat than had controls. Total fruit, vegetable, nuts, and whole grain intakes and olive oil consumption were also significantly higher in the intervention group. There were 13 men in the intervention group and 2 in the control group (P = .015) who reported an IIEF score of 22 or

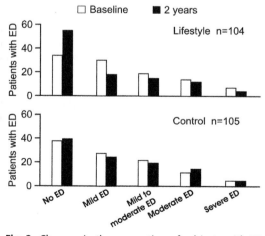

Fig. 2. Changes in the proportion of subjects with ED after randomization of 209 men to intensive lifestyle changes or control. No ED, score 22–25. In men assigned to lifestyle changes, there was a significant increase in the percentage of men without ED after the intervention.

higher. In the intervention group, changes in IIEF score were related to increased intake of fruits, vegetables, nuts, and legumes ($P<.01$) and the ratio of polyunsaturated to saturated lipids ($P<.02$).

The authors used the same protocol to study the effect of a Mediterranean-style diet on sexual function in women with the metabolic syndrome.[43] Thirty-one women with a diagnosis of FSD and metabolic syndrome were assigned to the Mediterranean-style diet and 28 to a standard control diet. After 2 years, women on the Mediterranean diet consumed more fruits, vegetables, nuts, whole grain, and olive oil compared with men on the control diet. FSFI improved in the intervention group, from a mean basal value of 19.7 $\pm$ 3.1 to a mean post-treatment value of 26.1 $\pm$ 4.1 ($P = .01$), and remained stable in the control group. No single sexual domain (desire, arousal, lubrication, orgasm, satisfaction, or pain) was significantly ameliorated by the dietary treatment, suggesting that the whole female sexuality may find benefit from lifestyle changes. A Mediterranean-style diet might be effective in ameliorating sexual function in women with the metabolic syndrome.

Lifestyle Recommendations for Sexual Problems

Major health organizations promote the adoption of a healthy lifestyle composed of sufficient daily physical activity and a balanced diet for the prevention and management CVD risk. In particular, it is recommended that adults accumulate 30 minutes of moderate-intensity aerobic physical activity on most days of the week. Despite these recommendations, a physically active lifestyle is seldom adopted, and the majority of the North American population remains sedentary. Current estimates suggest that more than half of Americans (51.9%)[44] perform less than the recommended minimum of 30 minutes of moderate-intensity physical activity on most days of the week. These statistics are alarming given that physical inactivity is a prominent risk factor for CVDs and along with poor nutrition is a leading cause of mortality in North America.[45]

Although the optimal strategy for promoting physical activity in today's environment remains elusive, the evidence for the utility of physical activity in the management of risk factors for CVD is overwhelming. Increases in physical activity levels are associated with clinically significant improvements in the following outcomes: visceral adiposity, insulin resistance, glucose homeostasis among diabetics, risk of type 2 diabetes mellitus among those at risk, high-density lipoprotein cholesterol, triglycerides, apolipoprotein B, blood pressure, inflammatory and thrombotic status, and cardiorespiratory fitness.[46] Changes in body composition rather than body weight are more meaningful outcomes in response to physical activity.[47] Significant reduction in fat mass, especially visceral fat, often occur concurrent with equal increases in lean body mass in response to physical activity. Nevertheless, although physical activity–induced weight loss is likely associated with the greatest reduction in visceral fat, it is equally important to recognize that visceral obesity can be markedly reduced in response to minimal weight loss.

Despite increased public awareness of the importance of diet in decreasing the risk of chronic disease, large gaps remain in food-based recommendations and actual dietary practice of the population. Swinburn and colleagues[48] postulated that increased obesity in the United States is attributed directly to increased food intake (ie, increased calorie consumption). The potential health benefits from reducing the prevalence of overweight—obesity in particular—are of significant public health importance, because excess bodyweight is the sixth most important risk factor contributing to death worldwide.[49] Data from the *National Health and Nutrition Examination Survey*[50] indicate that between 1971 and 2004, average total energy consumption among US adults increased by 22% in women (from 1542 to 1886 kcal/d) and by 10% in men (from 2450 to 2693 kcal/d). The increases in calories consumed during this time period are attributable primarily to greater average carbohydrate intake, in particular, of starches, refined grains, and sugars. Other specific changes related to increased caloric intake in the United States include larger portion sizes, greater food quantity and calories per meal, and increased consumption of sugar-sweetened beverages, snacks, commercially prepared (especially fast food) meals, and higher energy-density foods.

CURRENT LIMITATIONS AND FUTURE NEEDS

The low awareness of ED among men may be a shortcoming for a timely diagnosis of ED and may delay a comprehensive assessment of the overall cardiovascular risk in asymptomatic men. In 1053 men 30 years old and older presenting with at least one risk factor (controlled hypertension, hypercholesterolemia, smoking, metabolic syndrome, stable coronary artery disease, diabetes, depression, lower urinary tract symptoms, obesity, or waist circumference ≥ 40 inches) and without a diagnosis of ED, IIEF scores indicated ED occurred in 71% (744/1053). Only 139, however, were aware of their ED.[51] ED should be suspected

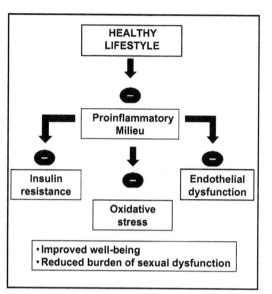

Fig. 3. Adoption of healthy lifestyles may reduce a proinflammatory milieu with a consequent amelioration of insulin sensitivity, endothelial functions, and oxidative stress. The resulting improved well-being may help contribute to reduce the burden of sexual dysfunctions in both genders.

and assessed in men with risk factors, regardless of their apparent level of awareness of ED.

A better understanding of what constitutes a normal sexual response in women would aid in improving the evaluation of efficacy. The female sexual response cycle is complex and dependent on physiologic, psychological, and social factors.[52] The complexity of the sexual response in women, including the relative independence between subjective and objective aspects of arousal and desire, makes it difficult to use a single measurement to evaluate efficacy. Recently completed randomized clinical trials have incorporated the use of the coprimary endpoints of change in satisfying sexual events and disorder-specific self-assessment questionnaires.

SUMMARY

A substantial body of knowledge demonstrates that adoption of healthy lifestyle, including consumption of healthy diets and increased physical activity, conveys a markedly lower risk of coronary disease.[29] The beneficial effect of healthy diets on atherosclerosis in general, and CHD in particular, can be mediated through multiple biologic pathways other than serum lipids, including reduction of oxidative stress and subclinical inflammation, amelioration of endothelial dysfunction and insulin sensitivity, and mitigation

of blood pressure and thrombotic tendency.[53–55] It could, therefore, be speculated that a healthy lifestyle may protect from chronic diseases that are related to low-grade subclinical inflammation, such as atherosclerosis and metabolic diseases, which are linked to ED in men. Promotion of a healthful lifestyle, including a healthy diet and exercise, for prevention and treatment among individuals at all ages yields great benefits and reduces the burden of chronic diseases; beyond the specific effects on sexual dysfunctions in both men and women, adoption of these measures promotes a healthier life and increased well being, which in turn may help to reduce the burden of sexual dysfunction (**Fig. 3**).

REFERENCES

1. Laumann EO, Paik A, Rosen RC. Sexual dysfunction in the United States: prevalence and predictors. JAMA 1999;281:537–44.
2. Ayta IA, McKinlay JB, Krane RJ. The likely worldwide increase in erectile dysfunction between 1995 and 2025 and some possible policy consequences. BJU Int 1999;84:50–6.
3. Feldman HA, Goldstein I, Hatzichristou DG, et al. Impotence and its medical and psychosocial correlates: results of the Massachusetts Male Aging Study. J Urol 1994;151:54–61.
4. O'Leary MP, Althof SE, Cappelleri JC, et al. Self-esteem, confidence and relationship satisfaction of men with erectile dysfunction treated with sildenafil citrate: a multicenter, randomized, parallel group, double-blind, placebo controlled study in the United States. J Urol 2006;175:1058–62.
5. McVary KT. Erectile dysfunction. N Engl J Med 2007; 357:2472–81.
6. Lue T, Basson R, Rosen R, et al. Sexual medicine. Sexual dysfunction in men and women. Second International consultation on sexual dysfunction. Paris: 2004 Health Publication; 2004.
7. Shifren JL, Monz BU, Russo PA, et al. Sexual problems and distress in United States women: prevalence and correlates. Obstet Gynecol 2008;112: 970–8.
8. Laumann EO, Nicolosi A, Glasser DB, et al. Sexual problems among women and men aged 40–80 y: prevalence and correlates identified in the Global Study of Sexual Attitudes and Behaviors. Int J Impot Res 2005;17:39–57.
9. Bacon CG, Mittleman MA, Kawachi I, et al. Sexual function in men older than 50 years of age: results from the health professionals follow-up study. Ann Intern Med 2003;139:161–8.
10. Larsen SH, Wagner G, Heitmann BL. Sexual function and obesity. Int J Obes (Lond) 2007;31:1189–98.

11. Feldman HA, Johannes CB, Derby CA, et al. Erectile dysfunction and coronary risk factors: prospective results from the Massachusetts Male Aging Study. Prev Med 2000;30:328–38.

12. Shiri R, Koskimäki J, Hakama M, et al. Effect of life-style factors on incidence of erectile dysfunction. Int J Impot Res 2004;16:389–94.

13. Fung MM, Bettencourt R, Barrett-Connor H. Heart disease risk factors predict erectile dysfunction 25 years later. J Am Coll Cardiol 2004;43:1405–11.

14. Adolfsson B, Elofsson S, Rossner S, et al. Are sexual dissatisfaction and sexual abuse associated with obesity? A population-based study. Obes Res 2004;12:1702–9.

15. Kolotkin RL, Binks M, Crosby RD, et al. Obesity and sexual quality of life. Obesity (Silver Spring) 2006; 14:472–9.

16. Esposito K, Ciotola M, Giugliano F, et al. Association of body weight with sexual function in women. Int J Impot Res 2007;19:353–7.

17. Cheng JY, Ng EM, Chen RY. Physical activity and erectile dysfunction: meta-analysis of population-based studies. Int J Impot Res 2007;19:245–52.

18. Kratzik CW, Lackner JE, Märk I, et al. How much physical activity is needed to maintain erectile function? Results of the Androx Vienna Municipality Study. Eur Urol 2009;55:509–16.

19. Lutfey KE, Link CL, Rosen RC, et al. Prevalence and correlates of sexual activity and function in women: results from the Boston Area Community Health (BACH) Survey. Arch Sex Behav 2009;38:514–27.

20. Gerber JR, Johnson JV, Bunn JY, et al. A longitudinal study of the effects of free testosterone and other psychosocial variables on sexual function during the natural traverse of menopause. Fertil Steril 2005;83:643–8.

21. Hess R, Conroy MB, Ness R, et al. Association of lifestyle and relationship factors with sexual functioning of women during midlife. J Sex Med 2009; 6:1358–68.

22. Esposito K, Maiorino MI, Bellastella G, et al. Determinants of female sexual dysfucntion in type 2 diabetes. Int J Impot Res 2010;22:179–84.

23. Bacon CG, Mittleman MA, Kawachi I, et al. A prospective study of risk factors for erectile dysfunction. J Urol 2006;176:217–21.

24. McCall-Hosenfeld JS, Freund KM, Legault C, et al. Sexual satisfaction and cardiovascular disease: the women's health initiative. Am J Med 2008;121: 295–301.

25. Kupelian V, Araujo AB, Chiu GR, et al. Relative contributions of modifiable risk factors to erectile dysfunction: results from the Boston Area Community Health (BACH) Survey. Prev Med 2010;50:19–25.

26. Chew KK, Bremner A, Stuckey B, et al. Alcohol consumption and male erectile dysfunction: an unfounded reputation for risk? J Sex Med 2009;6: 1386–94.

27. Cheng JY, Ng EM, Chen RY, et al. Alcohol consumption and erectile dysfunction: meta-analysis of population-based studies. Int J Impot Res 2007;19: 343–52.

28. Sullivan ME, Thompson CS, Dashwood MR, et al. Nitric oxide and penile erections: is erectile dysfunction another manifestation of vascular disease? Cardiovasc Res 1999;43:658–65.

29. Hu FB, Willett WC. Optimal diets for prevention of coronary heart disease. JAMA 2002;288: 2569–78.

30. Esposito K, Giugliano F, De Sio M, et al. Dietary factors in erectile dysfunction. Int J Impot Res 2006;18:370–4.

31. Giugliano F, Maiorino M, Bellastella G, et al. Adherence to mediterranean diet and erectile dysfunction in men with type 2 diabetes. J Sex Med 2010;7: 1911–7.

32. Giugliano F, Maiorino MI, Di Palo C, et al. Adherence to Mediterranean diet and sexual function in women with type 2 diabetes. J Sex Med 2010; 7:1883–90.

33. Esposito K, Giugliano F, Di Palo C, et al. Effect of lifestyle changes on erectile dysfunction in obese men: a randomized controlled trial. JAMA 2004; 291:2978–84.

34. Wing RR, Rosen RC, Fava JL, et al. Effects of weight loss intervention on erectile function in older men with type 2 diabetes in the Look AHEAD trial. J Sex Med 2010;7:156–65.

35. Esposito K, Ciotola M, Giugliano F, et al. Effects of intensive lifestyle changes on erectile dysfunction in men. J Sex Med 2009;6:243–50.

36. Kolotkin RL, Head S, Hamilton M, et al. Assessing impact of weight on quality of life. Obes Res 1995; 3:349–56.

37. Werlinger K, King TK, Clark MM, et al. Perceived changes in sexual functioning and body image following weight loss in an obese female population: a pilot study. J Sex Marital Ther 1997;23:74–8.

38. Kaukua J, Pekkarinen T, Sane T, et al. Sex hormones and sexual function in obese men losing weight. Obes Res 2003;11:689–94.

39. Kolotkin RL, Binks M, Crosby RD, et al. Improvements in sexual quality of life after moderate weight loss. Int J Impot Res 2008;20:487–92.

40. Khoo J, Piantadosi C, Worthley S, et al. Effects of a low-energy diet on sexual function and lower urinary tract symptoms in obese men. Int J Obes (Lond) 2010;34:1396–403.

41. White JR, Case DA, McWhirter D, et al. Enhanced sexual behavior in exercising men. Arch Sex Behav 1990;19:193–209.

42. Esposito K, Ciotola M, Giugliano F, et al. Mediterranean diet improves erectile function in subjects

with the metabolic syndrome. Int J Impot Res 2006; 18:405–10.

43. Esposito K, Ciotola M, Giugliano F, et al. Mediterranean diet improves sexual function in women with the metabolic syndrome. Int J Impot Res 2007;19: 486–91.

44. Centers for Disease Control and Prevention. U.S. Physical activity statistics. Washington, DC: Department of Health and Human Services; 2005.

45. Mokdad AH, Marks JS, Stroup DF, et al. Actual causes of death in the United States, 2000. JAMA 2004;291:1238–45.

46. Janiszewski PM, Ross R. The utility of physical activity in the management of global cardiometabolic risk. Obesity (Silver Spring) 2009;17(Suppl 3):S3–14.

47. Janiszewski PM, Ross R. Physical activity in the treatment of obesity: beyond body weight reduction. Appl Physiol Nutr Metab 2007;32:512–22.

48. Swinburn BA, Sacks G, Lo SK, et al. Estimating the changes in energy flux that characterize the rise in obesity prevalence. Am J Clin Nutr 2009; 89:1723–8.

49. Global health risks: mortality and burden of disease attributable to selected major risks. Geneve: WHO; 2009.

50. Roger VL, Go AS, Lloyd-Jones DM, et al. Heart disease and stroke statistics 2011 update: a report from the American Heart Association. Circulation 2011;123:e1–192.

51. Shabsigh R, Kaufman J, Magee M, et al. Lack of awareness of erectile dysfunction in many men with risk factors for erectile dysfunction. BMC Urol 2010;10:18.

52. Basson R. Female sexual response: the role of drugs in the management of sexual dysfunction. Obstet Gynecol 2001;98:350–3.

53. Lopez-Garcia E, Hu FB. Nutrition and the endothelium. Curr Diab Rep 2004;4:253–9.

54. Esposito K, Giugliano D. Diet and inflammation: a link to metabolic and cardiovascular disease. Eur Heart J 2006;27:15–20.

55. Giugliano D, Ceriello A, Esposito K. The effects of diet on inflammation: emphasis on the metabolic syndrome. J Am Coll Cardiol 2006;48:677–85.

Promoting Wellness for Patients on Androgen Deprivation Therapy: Why Using Numerous Drugs for Drug Side Effects Should Not Be First-Line Treatment

Mark A. Moyad, MD, MPH[a,b,*], Mack Roach III, MD[c]

KEYWORDS

• Androgen deprivation therapy • Prostate cancer
• Side effects • Toxicity

The controversy over androgen deprivation therapy (ADT) for prostate cancer seems to have shifted over the past decade. The issue of adverse events or side effects now seems to dominate over that of clinical efficacy in several scenarios.[1–3] A wide variety of side effects have been attributed either indirectly or directly to ADT in an acute or chronic situation, with little to no distinction as to whether the risk is novel, minimal, or highly prevalent.[4–7] This article is an update of a 2005 publication,[8] and provides an overview of some side effects attributed to ADT. However, the purpose is to provide evidence questioning the treatment of any, or most, of these side effects with numerous prescription medications that have their own unique toxicity profile. Select patients on ADT, rather than most, qualify for prescription medication to treat side effects. The efficacy of the drugs that are becoming increasingly popular for treating side effects of ADT is also compared with the efficacy of lifestyle changes, over-the-counter dietary supplementation, and some safe generic prescription agents.

ANEMIA

The anemia associated with ADT (continuous or intermittent) is usually the normochromic normocytic type (not microcytic or macrocytic),[9,10] which is somewhat similar to what is experienced in aging men,[11,12] except that it occurs within months in those undergoing ADT (acute) compared with decades in those experiencing normal aging (chronic). This acute reduction in hemoglobin occurs in most patients on ADT, with a mean of 10% or greater decrease in hemoglobin and red blood cell counts, but with minimal changes in mean corpuscular volume, and no changes in mean cell hemoglobin, mean cell hemoglobin concentration, or iron levels.[13] Thus, most patients with localized

[a] Department of Urology, University of Michigan Medical Center, 1500 East Medical Center Drive, Ann Arbor, MI 48109-0330, USA
[b] Eisenhower Wellness Institute, Eisenhower Medical Center, Rancho Mirage, CA, USA
[c] Department of Radiation Oncology, Helen Diller Family Comprehensive Cancer Center, University of California-San Francisco, 1600 Divisadero, 3rd Floor, San Francisco, CA 94115, USA
* Corresponding author. Department of Urology, University of Michigan Medical Center, 1500 East Medical Center Drive, Ann Arbor, MI 48109-0330.
E-mail address: moyad@umich.edu

Urol Clin N Am 38 (2011) 303–312
doi:10.1016/j.ucl.2011.05.001
0094-0143/11/$ – see front matter © 2011 Elsevier Inc. All rights reserved.

urologic.theclinics.com

or locally advanced or nonmetastatic prostate cancer do not require treatment with diet, dietary supplements (not iron, B_{12}, or folate), or prescription medications for this side effect. If ADT is discontinued, the anemia should dissipate with testosterone normalization. Therefore, just as excessive testosterone levels or testosterone replacement therapy can lead to polycythemia,[14] minimal testosterone levels can lead to anemia. Some preliminary evidence suggests that the hemoglobin changes on average are lower in men without bone metastasis who perform regular resistance exercises.[15] In patients with metastasis, anemia is more likely to become symptomatic during ADT treatment, and some of these individuals may require conventional drug treatment.[16]

BONE AND MUSCLE LOSS

The predicted risk of bone loss may be exaggerated in contemporary patients on ADT because older data are being used. These older studies do not take into account that patients are now more preventive-minded and informed, and use methods to avoid this risk. Older studies involved patients with more advanced disease who were usually not on minimal forms of preventive therapy for bone loss, and yearly rates of spinal bone loss were reported to be as high as 5% to 8.5%, and as much as 2% to 6.5% in the hip.[17] However, research on Japanese patients with prostate cancer found a low rate of osteoporosis (approximately 10%–12%).[18,19] Patients treated with ADT have significantly reduced bone mineral density (BMD) numbers and T scores and z scores compared with hormone-naïve Japanese patients, but research continues to show no significant increase of osteoporosis prevalence in these men who had been on ADT for a mean of 30.7 months. Heart-healthy lifestyle changes common among the older Japanese population may contribute to this finding.[20]

Additionally, calcium and vitamin D deficiencies and a lack of resistance activity are some of the many factors that can lead to a misrepresentation of the true rate of bone loss associated with ADT. More recent research conducted in the United States and internationally has suggested a reduced risk of bone loss in men receiving calcium and vitamin D supplementation while on ADT[21,22]; unfortunately, only a minority (10%–20%) of patients are following these simplistic recommendations, largely because of a lack of education from their providers.[22–25]

Perhaps if the playing field were leveled in terms of comparing pharmacologic bone preservation therapy with lifestyle changes and supplements in patients with nonmetastatic disease on ADT, this might provide an unbiased assessment of the true need for pharmacologic treatment of this condition. Few older studies have addressed this issue, with some exceptions, including two studies of zoledronic acid in patients with nonmetastatic disease. In these studies, the placebo intervention involved a calcium supplement at a low, inadequate dose (500 mg) and vitamin D intakes of 400 to 500 IU. A rate of bone loss of 2% to 3% was seen in 12 months at the major anatomic sites of interest (spine and hip).[26,27] In the first study, no participant experienced a clinical or symptomatic fracture, but five new or exacerbated vertebral fractures were diagnosed on imaging in the zoledronic acid group versus three in the placebo group.[26] In the second study, results were similar in terms of fracture incidence, and especially in BMD changes, which were not as excessive as older reports, perhaps because the supplementation in the placebo group was at least minimal.[27] These two studies were too short to report or observe fractures, so little focus was placed on fracture differences, but the lack of fractures should still be of interest to the reader.

Two other studies, one with a weekly oral[28] and another with a 6-month injectable pharmacologic medication, also provide insight into this issue.[29] A randomized 1-year trial of 112 men with nonmetastatic prostate cancer on ADT compared weekly oral alendronate with placebo.[28] Both arms of the study received calcium carbonate with vitamin D (each tablet has 500 mg of calcium and 200 IU of vitamin D) to ensure a total calcium intake greater than 1000 mg/d. At baseline, median duration on ADT was 14 months, and vitamin D levels were greater than 30 ng/mL. BMD changes at the spine were −1.4% for the placebo group, −0.7% at the femoral neck, and −1.8% at the distal radius. One fracture occurred in each group. However, despite no T score differences in the spine among the groups (−0.26), hip BMD and other hip anatomic sites were significantly lower at baseline in the placebo arm, as were measurements at the distal third of the radius.

Furthermore, significantly more patients ($P = .02$) in the placebo group had osteopenia or osteoporosis (95% vs 88%). A total of 52% of patients at baseline had osteoporosis compared with 27% treated with the oral drug. Had the participants been able to perform regular resistance exercises and institute heart-healthy lifestyle changes before initiating ADT, it would have been interesting to observe whether any noticeable or tangible differences could be seen between the arms.

Another relevant study involved the use of the recently published, large, 3-year trial of denosumab given every 6 months (n = 734) compared with placebo (n = 734) in men receiving ADT for nonmetastatic prostate cancer.[29] All of the participants were instructed take 1000 mg or more of calcium and 400 IU of vitamin D. This trial represents one of the first long-term randomized studies to provide the placebo arm with realistic and relevant dietary supplementation. Median serum vitamin D levels at baseline were 24 to 25 ng/mL, and increased to 31 ng/mL (normal range) after 36 months. Mean T score was similar in this study compared with the previous study (–0.3), but only 14% to 15% of participants began the trial with osteoporosis (T score <–2.5) at any site, compared with 52% in the placebo arm of the previous trial. Thus, these patients had less-severe bone loss overall compared with the previous study, despite the longer median time on ADT at a baseline of 20 to 21 months.

The primary end point was the percent change in BMD at the lumbar spine at 24 months, and secondary end points included percent change in BMD at the femoral neck and total hip at 24 months, and at all three anatomic locations at 36 months, along with incidence of new fractures. After 24 months a significant loss in lumbar spine BMD was seen in the placebo group, but the actual loss was only 1%, and minimally changed at 36 months. Significant reductions in femoral neck and total hip were also seen, but these losses were only 2% to 3% at 36 months. The largest loss occurred in the distal radius. Incidence of fracture at any anatomic location was lower with denosumab than with placebo, but the difference was not found to be statistically significant at 36 months.

Furthermore, no significant differences were found in the time to first fracture (nonvertebral or vertebral) between the groups. The authors reported that more than one fracture at any location occurred in significantly more patients on placebo than denosumab, and that these patients also had a significantly higher rate of vertebral fractures. However, these are secondary end points, and more participants in the placebo group had a history of vertebral fracture (+2.6%) and osteoporotic fracture (+4.5%) at baseline. The 36-month clinical difference of 2.4% more new vertebral fractures (3.9% vs 1.5%) in the placebo group cannot be fully attributed to the intervention itself, but may also have been from the inequality between groups in terms of vertebral and overall fractures at baseline in favor of denosumab. In other words, the differences between most clinical end points for the calcium and vitamin D group compared with pharmacologic treatment was, in the authors' opinion, minimal at 36 months. Furthermore, a less than 4% total fracture percentage in the placebo arm (vs 1.9%) over 3 years is low considering that these patients did not make aggressive lifestyle changes or take supplemental preventive therapy before ADT was initiated. Again, this leaves one to ponder how much difference would have really been seen if the placebo group were also assigned to regular resistance and aerobic exercises during this study period or before initiating ADT, interventions that in small studies have been able to maintain BMD alone without supplementation.[15]

Perhaps the most interesting benefit of denosumab may be in men who cannot adequately maintain distal radius density with aggressive lifestyle changes. A slightly higher rate of serious adverse events with denosumab (34.6% vs 30.6%) was also observed in the ADT trial,[29] and an accompanying editorial expressed concerns raised in other studies about a potential negative impact on the immune system.[30] Emerging evidence also has shown that this drug can cause the rare side effect of osteonecrosis of the jaw, and hypocalcemia is not uncommon.[31] Regardless, little doubt exists that preventing osteoporosis with pharmacologic agents such as denosumab in patients with castration-resistant prostate cancer can have a profound impact on skeletal-related events, and the potential increases in radial bone mineral density with this drug cannot be matched by other less-aggressive interventions.[31] However, early use of these drugs in patients without metastasis who are about to begin ADT rather than implement lifestyle changes, supplements (calcium and vitamin D), and resistance exercise should be at least questioned.

When reviewing the data from the four trials of pharmacologic intervention in patients without metastasis, several observations should be considered.[26–29] As investigators used more appropriate supplementation of calcium and normalization of vitamin D status during the last two pharmacologic trials[28,29] compared with the first two,[26,27] reductions in bone loss at the major anatomic sites were progressively less in the placebo arms, and perhaps even stabilized after 1 year (eg, at the lumbar spine, the primary end point of the denosumab trial).[29] Again, this treatment was given without encouraging regular aerobic and resistance exercise, suggesting that a clinical trial of patients without metastasis on ADT with adequate calcium and vitamin D status with aerobic and resistance exercise may compare favorably to pharmacologic intervention over 1 year or more.

Another important factor is that denosumab and zoledronic acid trials have used low to moderate amounts of calcium and vitamin D to enhance the efficacy of the drug itself.[31] Thus, clinicians should encourage calcium and vitamin D supplements in patients on ADT regardless of their bone-preserving drug treatment status. Perhaps more appropriately, they should have the patient meet with a nutritionist to determine their average calcium intake from food, and not exceed the daily 1200 mg requirement with a supplement, regardless of low or average calcium food intake.[32] Furthermore, vitamin D status should be normalized through using approximately 1000 IU/d of vitamin D, and monitoring 25(OH)-vitamin D status to ensure proper levels (30–40 ng/mL or 75–100 nmol/L). Preliminary evidence suggests that daily use of vitamin D supplementation may be more effective at increasing vitamin D serum status than equivalent oral dosing weekly or monthly.[33]

Sarcopenia is simply a progressive reduction in skeletal muscle mass, strength, and quality, and, in some cases, the replacement of these anatomic sites by adipose tissue, which not only occurs with aging but also is accelerated by ADT at upper and lower body sites.[34,35] Clinical research is also beginning to emerge that sarcopenia can actually improve significantly if men on ADT perform upper and lower body resistance exercises at least twice a week, regardless of the time on ADT.[36] No drug has been able to accomplish these results. Patients must be informed that the only consistent proven treatment for preventing sarcopenia with aging, or during ADT, is regular resistance and aerobic exercise, which also promote heart health.[36,37] Furthermore, the reductions in skeletal muscle mass and contractile properties with sarcopenia is also associated with increases in insulin resistance, lipids, and fat tissue.[37] Theoretically, the benefits of regular and perhaps even more-intensive resistance activity in men and women could outweigh the benefits of calcium and vitamin D supplementation, as was recently found in a randomized trial of men without prostate cancer.[38] Regardless, clinicians must determine whether the harm outweighs the benefits when beginning a resistance exercise program in a patient who has metastatic disease.

Novel simplistic interventions to combat sarcopenia that could be independently or synergistically beneficial along with resistance activity have been known for some time but not used or encouraged with ADT.[39,40] For example, because vitamin D receptors are found on muscle tissue, older individuals with normal vitamin D status seem to have a lower risk of sarcopenia.[41] Calcium supplementation may also have this impact for a similar reason, and the combined synergism may reduce the risk of falls.[32] Higher dietary protein intakes beyond the standard, which is currently 0.8 g/kg/d (regardless of age) may stimulate muscle protein synthesis and is safe.[42–44]

Intakes of 1.0 to 1.2, and even 1.5 g/kg/d of protein in some cases (20% of total caloric intake), may benefit older individuals with sarcopenia or may prevent its development. This practice could also favorably impact calcium absorption to improve BMD, maintain nitrogen balance, and avoid compromising renal function.

One of the most interesting, novel, and evolving approaches for preventing sarcopenia is high-quality but diverse amino acid or protein supplementation via low-calorie powders, capsules, or liquids. For example, clinical studies in elderly people have already documented increased lean body mass, reduction in fat mass, and increased handgrip strength, leg strength, and muscle protein synthesis with essential amino acid supplementation for several months.[45–48] Because small increases in insulin-like growth factor 1 can also occur with protein supplementation (similar to resistance exercise), more research should be conducted on patients with cancer using these interventions, but the overall health benefit seems to trump any specific physiologic concern. The authors believe this is tantamount to the original concern and subsequent debunking of the myth that resistance exercise can exacerbate lymphedema in breast cancer.[49] Additionally, far more concerning interventions in patients with prostate cancer, such as dehydroepiandrosterone supplementation and growth hormone replacement, have failed to provide tangible benefits in elderly patients.[50,51] In fact, one of the most interesting older studies of growth hormone supplementation found no added benefit, especially in elderly patients engaged in strength training via resistance exercise first for 14 weeks before supplementing with this hormone.[52] Clinicians should promote more heart-healthy and cost-effective interventions that are more promising. For example, fish oil is another supplement that has recently garnered new data regarding sarcopenia prevention through potentially reducing some inflammatory markers.[53]

CHOLESTEROL/LIPID CHANGES/CARDIOVASCULAR DISEASE

Much controversy and debate has centered on whether ADT increases the risk of cardiovascular disease events or mortality, or negatively impacts all-cause mortality.[54] Some retrospective and prospective data suggest that it does,[54] but randomized controlled trials have not found a consistent significant increase in risk, and recent trials even suggest a benefit.[55–57] Additionally, research suggests that ADT can increase weight, glucose, triglycerides,[58] and low-density lipoproteins (LDLs), but paradoxically it also increases high-density lipoproteins

(HDLs) or Apo-A, which are markers for cardiovascular disease prevention.[59,60]

Regardless of the side of the argument, one observation that needs little discussion is that cardiovascular disease is either the number one or two potential cause of death in men, those with prostate cancer, or those on ADT.[8] Thus, all men on ADT still should attempt to reduce their cardiovascular disease risk as much as possible. A combination of lifestyle changes, fish oil supplementation, and a low-dose statin could arguably provide this type of needed protection during ADT. One of the most relevant studies comparing men on ADT with and without the use of statins found significant increases in HDL and the prevention of a significant increase in LDL for men on statins, but still showed a significant increase in triglycerides.[61] Perhaps the concern of weight gain and triglyceride increases should also be addressed, beyond lifestyle changes and statins in men on ADT.

Fish oil is approved the US Food and Drug Administration for lowering triglycerides, and some consistent data suggest that it may lower the risk of insulin resistance,[62–67] but this has not been studied in patients on ADT. However, some clinical data suggest a reduction in the incidence of diabetes in patients with ADT on vitamin D.[68] The American Heart Association recommends a daily intake of 1000 mg of the main components of fish oil (EPA and DHA) in individuals with heart disease, and the inclusion of plant sources of omega-3s,[69] and it could be argued that this should potentially include patients on ADT. A large randomized trial combining statins with 1800 mg of EPA (found in fish oil supplements) in individuals with high cholesterol found synergistic benefits in healthy men and women.[70]

The Japanese JELIS trial randomized 9326 participants to a total of 1800 mg of fish oil (600 mg three times daily after meals) and 10 to 20 mg of pravastatin or 5 to 10 mg of simvastatin (both generic statin and cost-effective) daily, and compared them with a control group of 9319 participants on statin treatment alone. After a mean of only 4.6 years, fish oil significantly reduced unstable angina (0.76; $P = .01$), nonfatal coronary events (0.81; $P = .015$), and the primary end point of major coronary events (0.81; $P = .01$). This trial showed that omega-3 supplementation could provide a synergistic impact for patients on statin treatment. Furthermore, the fish consumption of the participants was already adequate or beyond moderate, but supplementation still provided benefits. No differences were found in total cholesterol, LDL, or HDL between groups, but triglycerides were significantly reduced in the fish oil group compared with controls (–9% vs –4%; $P<.001$). A recent subanalysis of the JELIS trial found that participants with impaired glucose metabolism who were taking fish oil had a significant reduction (–22%) in coronary artery disease incidence that was even greater than the significant reduction in normoglycemic (–18%) individuals.[71] Resistance exercise also reduces glucose or more favorably controls insulin in patients on ADT and other individuals,[36,37] and it significantly improved triglycerides in another clinical trial of patients on ADT also receiving radiation therapy.[72] It could be argued that triglycerides, glucose, and insulin sensitivity will improve in most patients on ADT with an increase in muscle mass or reduction in body fat, because triglycerides are stored in adipose tissue, and metabolism is further reduced with declining muscle mass.[8,37]

FATIGUE, HOT FLASHES, AND MENTAL HEALTH

Fatigue was significantly reduced in a 12-week randomized trial of aerobic and resistance exercise in patients on ADT.[36] Increases in muscle mass, metabolism, and energy levels were also noted.[37] Another large randomized trial of American ginseng (panax quinquefolius) compared with placebo found a potential reduction in reported fatigue among patients with cancer assigned to 1000 or 2000 mg/d of this herbal compound.[73] Side effects were similar to those of placebo.

Treatments for hot flashes are arguably more extensively studied in breast cancer than any other tumor type.[74,75] Perhaps the lessons learned should be applied to the prostate carcinoma research, including the use of a hot flash diary for patients in clinical studies and clinical practice. Recently, one trial involving patients with prostate cancer addressed pharmacologic interventions compared with nonintervention in men on ADT with hot flashes.[76] A total of 311 men who had already received 6 months of ADT were randomly assigned to one of three regimens daily for 12 weeks: 75 mg of venlafaxine, 100 mg of cyproterone acetate, or 20 mg of medroxyprogesterone acetate. Patients also completed a 1-week hot flash diary before each clinical visit. Participants included in the analysis reported that 80% of their hot flashes on average were moderate to severe before the randomization period (using a hot flash diary at home to assess vasomotor symptoms). The change in median hot flash score was –47% for venlafaxine, –94% for cyproterone, and –84% for medroxyprogesterone, and the decrease was significant ($P<.0001$) for each medication from baseline, but a significant improvement was seen for

Table 1
Lifestyle changes and other minimal interventions to prevent and treat the side effects of androgen deprivation therapy

Lifestyle Changes and/or Dietary Supplement	Potential Benefit While on ADT
Aerobic exercise every other day, and weight lifting/resistance exercise just 2–3 times a week (note: metastatic disease patients may not qualify for weight lifting because of a potential increased risk of fracture)	Improves heart and mental health Reduces bone loss Reduces weight gain May improve anemia Reduces bone loss Reduces sarcopenia Reduces fatigue Improves cardiovascular health
Heart-healthy diet (eg, Mediterranean diet)	Improves heart and mental health
Aspirin	May improve heart health in those at high risk May reduce inflammatory markers
Calcium and vitamin D supplementation	Reduces bone loss May reduce risk of insulin insensitivity
Cholesterol lowering (statin or over-the-counter statin equivalent, such as red yeast rice extract)	Reduces risk of elevated low-density lipoprotein and triglycerides Reduces inflammatory markers May promote bone health
Diary	Record number and intensity of hot flashes Record any other issues with ADT and provide this record to physician
Fish oil and plant sources of omega-3 fatty acids	Reduces triglycerides May reduce insulin resistance May reduce sarcopenia May reduce hot flash frequency
Ginseng (Panax quinquefolius)	May reduce fatigue
Protein or amino acid powder supplementation	May reduce sarcopenia with resistance activity May improve calcium absorption May reduce weight gain May reduce fatigue by maintaining muscle mass

cyproterone and medroxyprogesterone over venlafaxine. Furthermore, approximately one-quarter to one-third of hot flashes in these two groups were eliminated. The authors concluded that medroxyprogesterone should be considered the standard treatment for hot flashes in men on ADT that need treatment, because cyproterone is a treatment for prostate cancer that could interfere with ADT.

However, another interesting observation was made in this trial.[76] A total of only 22% of men that had received ADT for 6 months actually spontaneously requested hot flash treatment, which caused difficulty in recruiting to the trial. In other words, only approximately one of every five men either felt they needed hot flash pharmacologic treatment or requested it. Based on this observation, the authors commented directly that, "In our view, this justifies the recommendation not to systematically prevent hot flashes in all patients on initiation of an androgen-suppressing treatment."[76]

Arguably, this finding suggests that men should use a diary and, based on the results, clinicians should discuss the need for lifestyle or pharmacologic intervention in case patients do not have knowledge about treatment or are not comfortable discussing the subject.

Another interesting observation from this study was the significant benefit on the emotional functional scale that only occurred in patients in the venlafaxine arm and appeared early in the study (within 4 weeks).[76] This benefit should be construed as another reason to individualize treatment for ADT side effects and consider treating men with a need for mental and emotional improvement on ADT and experiencing moderate to severe hot flashes with venlafaxine, or another similar class medication compared with progesterone.

Based on past studies, little doubt exists overall that progesterone treatments (megestrol acetate pills or medroxyprogesterone depot injections or pills) are among the most effective and least costly pharmacologic treatments available for men with moderate to severe hot flashes.[76,77] However, progesterone is not without potential issues at higher doses, including adipose tissue increases, HDL reduction, appetite stimulation, sarcopenia acceleration, fatigue, and sexual dysfunction.[78,79] All of these issues are added to the ongoing ADT issues, and should provide enough reason to be judicious in its use.

Indirect clinical evidence for fish oil suggests potential in reducing hot flash frequency (not intensity) and improving mental health.[80–82]

SUMMARY

The lifestyle, supplement, and even statin interventions promoted in this article are heart-healthy with minimal risk of serious adverse events, and could provide multiple diverse benefits for patients on ADT. **Table 1** summarizes the potential benefits, which could be given as a handout to patients to encourage them to follow this program. Additionally, the beneficial research on heart-healthy supplementation and lifestyle changes is still in initial stages, and the possibilities seem limitless in terms of what side effects can be prevented or controlled. For example, emerging heart-healthy research suggests that lipid-lowering or omega-3 interventions may provide bone health benefits and even survival benefits, or that protein powder or fish oil supplementation may control weight gain.[83–88] Even the recent data on low-dose or regular aspirin show that patients who qualify may receive ancillary anticancer benefits,[8,89,90] but a more careful assessment by clinicians should be performed, because for some patients the risk of adverse events could exceed the benefit.[91]

The hope is that the days of patients being considered passive participants in the prevention and treatment of ADT side effects are gone. Clinicians and patients are now replete with information that could potentially mitigate most side effects of ADT. However, trading one type of toxicity from ADT for another potential toxicity from ADT prescription medications, or even supplements, with the goal of preventing or treating side effects of cancer treatment does not seem to be advantageous, but rather a lateral step in medicine. Several patients on ADT clearly can greatly benefit from prescription medications of all kinds, especially those with metastatic disease. However, it is also recognized that the use of these medications may be embellished or exaggerated and based on older data that did not have access to novel simplistic preventive information on side effects. Promoting wellness

is tantamount to recommending heart-healthy lifestyle changes, supplements, and noninvasive medications for patients on ADT to reduce the number one and two cause of morbidity and mortality in these men. The authors believe that promoting this "forest over the isolated tree" approach increases the probability, more than most other interventions, that men on ADT will improve the quality and quantity of their life.

REFERENCES

1. Sharifi N, Gulley JL, Dahut WL. An update on androgen therapy for prostate cancer. Endocr Relat Cancer 2010;17:R305–15.
2. Wilson AC, Meethal SV, Bowen RL, et al. Leuprolide acetate: a drug of diverse clinical applications. Expert Opin Investig Drugs 2007;16:1851–63.
3. Mottet N, Bellmunt J, Bolla M, et al. EAU guidelines on prostate cancer. Part II: treatment of advanced, relapsing, and castration-resistant prostate cancer. Eur Urol 2011;59:572–83.
4. Adler RA. Management of osteoporosis in men on androgen deprivation therapy. Maturitas 2011;68: 143–7.
5. Beebe-Dimmer J, Morgenstern H, Cetin K, et al. Androgen deprivation therapy and cataract incidence among elderly prostate cancer patients in the United States. Ann Epidemiol 2011;21:156–63.
6. Kim HS, Freedland SJ. Androgen deprivation therapy in prostate cancer: anticipated side-effects and their management. Curr Opin Support Palliat Care 2010;4:147–52.
7. Saylor PJ, Keating NL, Smith MR. Prostate cancer survivorship: prevention and treatment of the adverse effects of androgen deprivation therapy. J Gen Intern Med 2009;24(Suppl 2):S389–94.
8. Moyad MA. Promoting general health during androgen deprivation therapy (ADT): a rapid 10-step review for your patients. Urol Oncol 2005;23:56–64.
9. Strum SB, McDermed JE, Scholz MC, et al. Anaemia associated with androgen deprivation in patients with prostate cancer receiving combined hormone blockade. Br J Urol 1997;79:933–41.
10. Malone S, Perry G, Segal R, et al. Long-term side-effects of intermittent androgen suppression therapy in prostate cancer: results of a phase II study. BJU Int 2005;96:514–20.
11. Nilsson-Ehle H, Jagenburg R, Landahl S, et al. Blood hemoglobin declines in the elderly: implications for reference intervals from age 70 to 88. Eur J Haematol 2000;65:297–305.
12. Ferrucci L, Maggio M, Bandinelli S, et al. Low testosterone levels and the risk of anemia in older men and women. Arch Intern Med 2006;166:1380–8.
13. Hara N, Nishiyama T, Takizawa I, et al. Decline of the red blood cell count in patients receiving androgen

deprivation therapy for localized prostate cancer: impact of ADT on insulin-like growth factor-1 and erythropoiesis. Urology 2010;75:1441–5.

14. Borst SE, Mulligan T. Testosterone replacement therapy for older men. Clin Interv Aging 2007;2:561–6.

15. Galvao DA, Nosaka K, Taaffe DR, et al. Resistance training and reduction of treatment side effects in prostate cancer patients. Med Sci Sports Exerc 2006;38:2045–52.

16. Curtis KK, Adam TJ, Chen SC, et al. Anaemia following initiation of androgen deprivation therapy for metastatic prostate cancer: a retrospective chart review. Aging Male 2008;11:157–61.

17. Diamond TH, Higan CS, Smith MR, et al. Osteoporosis in men with prostate carcinoma receiving androgen-deprivation therapy: recommendations for diagnosis and therapies. Cancer 2004;100:892–9.

18. Wang W, Yussa T, Tsuchiya N, et al. Bone mineral density in Japanese prostate cancer patients under androgen-deprivation therapy. Endocr Relat Cancer 2008;15:943–52.

19. Yuasa T, Maita S, Tsuchiya N, et al. Relationship between bone mineral density and androgen-deprivation therapy in Japanese prostate cancer patients. Urology 2010;75:1131–7.

20. Iso H. Lifestyle and cardiovascular disease in Japan. J Atheroscler Thromb 2011;18:83–8.

21. Ryan CW, Huo D, Stallings JW, et al. Lifestyle factors and duration of androgen deprivation affect bone mineral density of patients with prostate cancer during first year of therapy. Urology 2007;70:122–6.

22. Planas J, Morote J, Orsola A, et al. The relationship between daily calcium intake and bone mineral density in men with prostate cancer. BJU Int 2007;99:812–5.

23. Wilcox A, Carnes ML, Moon TD, et al. Androgen deprivation in veterans with prostate cancer: implications for skeletal health. Ann Pharmacother 2006; 40:2107–14.

24. Panju AH, Breunis H, Cheung AM, et al. Management of decreased bone mineral density in men starting androgen-deprivation therapy for prostate cancer. BJU Int 2009;103:753–7.

25. Yee EF, White RE, Murata GH, et al. Osteoporosis management in prostate cancer patients treated with androgen deprivation therapy. J Gen Intern Med 2007;22:1305–10.

26. Smith MR, Eastham J, Gleason D, et al. Randomized controlled trial of zoledronic acid to prevent bone loss in men receiving androgen deprivation therapy for nonmetastatic prostate cancer. J Urol 2003;169: 2008–12.

27. Ryan CW, Huo D, Demers LM, et al. Zoledronic acid initiated during the first year of androgen deprivation therapy increases bone mineral density in patients with prostate cancer. J Urol 2006;176:972–8.

28. Greenspan SL, Nelson JB, Trump DL, et al. Effect of once-weekly oral alendronate on bone loss in men

29. Smith MR, Egerdie B, Harnandez Toriz N, et al. Denosumab in men receiving androgen-deprivation therapy for prostate cancer. N Engl J Med 2009; 361:745–55.

30. Khosla S. Increasing options for the treatment of osteoporosis. N Engl J Med 2009;361:818–20.

31. Fizazi K, Carducci M, Smith M, et al. Denosumab versus zoledronic acid for treatment of bone metastases in men with castration-resistant prostate cancer: a randomized, double-blind study. Lancet 2011;377:813–22.

32. Reid IR, Ames R, Mason B, et al. Randomized controlled trial of calcium supplementation in healthy, nonosteoporotic, older men. Arch Intern Med 2008;168:2276–82.

33. Chel V, Wijnhoven HA, Smit JH, et al. Efficacy of different doses and time intervals of oral vitamin D supplementation with or without calcium in elderly nursing home residents. Osteoporos Int 2008;19:663–71.

34. Galvao DA, Spry NA, Taaffe DR, et al. Changes in muscle, fat and bone mass after 36 weeks of maximal androgen blockade for prostate cancer. BJU Int 2008;102:44–7.

35. Galvao DA, Taaffe DR, Spry N, et al. Reduced muscle strength and functional performance in men with prostate cancer undergoing androgen suppression: a comprehensive cross-sectional investigation. Prostate Cancer Prostatic Dis 2009;12:198–203.

36. Galvao DA, Taaffe DR, Spry N, et al. Combined resistance and aerobic exercise program reverses muscle loss in men undergoing androgen suppression therapy for prostate cancer without bone metastases: a randomized controlled trial. J Clin Oncol 2010;28:340–7.

37. Braith RW, Stewart KJ. Resistance exercise training: its role in the prevention of cardiovascular disease. Circulation 2006;113:2642–50.

38. Kukuljan S, Nowson CA, Sanders KM, et al. Independent and combined effects of calcium-vitamin d3 and exercise on bone structure and strength in older men: an 18-month factorial design randomized controlled trial. J Clin Endocrinol Metab 2011;96: 955–63.

39. Roubenoff R. Sarcopenia: a major modifiable cause of frailty in the elderly. J Nutr Health Aging 2000;4: 140–2.

40. von Haehling S, Morley JE, Anker SD. An overview of sarcopenia: facts and numbers on prevalence and clinical impact. J Cachex Sarcopenia Muscle 2010; 1:129–33.

41. Scott D, Blizzard L, Fell J, et al. A prospective study of the associations between 25-hydroxy-vitamin D, sarcopenia progression and physical activity in older adults. Clin Endocrinol 2010;73:581–7.

42. Wolfe RR, Miller SL, Miller KB. Optimal protein intake in the elderly. Clin Nutr 2008;27:675–84.

43. Wolfe RR, Miller SL. The recommended dietary allowance of protein: a misunderstood concept. JAMA 2008;299:2891–3.

44. Gaffney-Stomberg E, Insogna KL, Rodriguez NR, et al. Increasing dietary protein requirements in elderly people for optimal muscle and bone health. J Am Geriatr Soc 2009;57:1073–9.

45. Borsheim E, Bui QU, Tissier S, et al. Effect of amino acid supplementation on muscle mass, strength and physical function in the elderly. Clin Nutr 2008;27: 189–95.

46. Scognamiglio R, Avogaro A, Negut C, et al. The effects of oral amino acid intake on ambulatory capacity in elderly subjects. Aging Clin Exp Res 2004;16:443–7.

47. Dillon EL, Sheffield-Moore M, Paddon-Jones D, et al. Amino acid supplementation increases lean body mass, basal muscle protein synthesis, and insulin-like growth factor-I expression in older women. J Clin Endocrinol Metab 2009;94(5):1630–7.

48. Pennings B, Boirie Y, Senden JM, et al. Whey protein stimulates postprandial muscle protein accretion more effectively than do casein and casein hydroly-sate in older men. Am J Clin Nutr 2011;93:997–1005.

49. Schmitz KH, Ahmed RL, Troxel AB, et al. Weight lift-ing for women at risk for breast cancer-related lym-phedema: a randomized trial. JAMA 2010;304: 2699–705.

50. Nair KS, Rizza RA, O'Brien P, et al. DHEA in elderly women and DHEA or testosterone in elderly men. N Engl J Med 2006;355:1647–59.

51. Blackman MR, Sorkin JD, Munzer T, et al. Growth hormone and sex steroid administration in healthy aged women and men: a randomized controlled trial. JAMA 2002;288:2282–92.

52. Taaffe DR, Pruitt L, Reim J, et al. Effect of recombi-nant growth hormone on the muscle strength response to resistance exercise in elderly men. J Clin Endocrinol Metab 1994;79:1361–6.

53. Smith GI, Atherton P, Reeds DN, et al. Dietary omega-3 fatty acid supplementation increases the rate of muscle protein synthesis in older adults: a randomized controlled trial. Am J Clin Nutr 2011; 93:402–12.

54. Levine GN, D'Amico AV, Berger P, et al. Androgen-deprivation therapy in prostate cancer and cardio-vascular risk: a science advisory from the American Heart Association, American Cancer Society, and American Urological Association: endorsed by the American Society for Radiation Oncology. Circula-tion 2010;121:833–40.

55. Efstathiou JA, Bae K, Shipley WU, et al. Cardiovas-cular mortality and duration of androgen deprivation for locally advanced prostate cancer: analysis of RTOG 92-02. Eur Urol 2008;54:816–23.

56. Roach M 3rd, Bae K, Speight J, et al. Short-term neoadjuvant androgen deprivation therapy and external-beam radiotherapy for locally advanced prostate cancer: long-term results of RTOG 8610. J Clin Oncol 2008;26:585–91.

57. Denham JW, Steigler A, Lamb DS, et al. Short-term neoadjuvant androgen deprivation and radiotherapy for locally advanced prostate cancer: 10-year data from the TROG 96.01 randomised trial. Lancet On-col 2011;12(5):451–9.

58. Haseen F, Murray LJ, Cardwell CR, et al. The effect of androgen deprivation therapy on body composi-tion in men with prostate cancer: systematic review and meta-analysis. J Cancer Surviv 2010;4:128–39.

59. Smith MR, Lee H, McGovern F, et al. Metabolic changes during gonadotropin-releasing hormone agonist therapy for prostate cancer: differences from the classic metabolic syndrome. Cancer 2008;112:2188–94.

60. Eri LM, Urdal P, Bechensteen AG. Effects of the lutei-nizing hormone-releasing hormone agonist leupro-lide on lipoproteins, fibrinogen and plasminogen activator inhibitor in patients with benign prostatic hyperplasia. J Urol 1995;154:100–4.

61. Yannucci J, Manola J, Garnick MB, et al. The effect of androgen deprivation therapy on fasting serum lipid and glucose parameters. J Urol 2006;176:520–5.

62. Fetterman JW Jr, Zdanowicz MM. Therapeutic potential of n-3 polyunsaturated fatty acids in disease. Am J Health Syst Pharm 2009;66:1169–79.

63. Taouis M, Dagou C, Ster C, et al. N-3 polyunsatu-rated fatty acids prevent the defect of insulin receptor signaling in muscle. Am J Physiol Endocri-nol Metab 2002;282:E664–71.

64. Lombardo YB, Chicco AG. Effects of dietary polyun-saturated n-3 fatty acids on dyslipidemia and insulin resistance in rodents and humans. A review. J Nutr Biochem 2006;17:1–13.

65. Fedor D, Kelley DS. Prevention of insulin resistance by n-3 polyunsaturated fatty acids. Curr Opin Clin Nutr Metab Care 2009;12:138–46.

66. Carpenter YA, Portois L, Malaisse WJ. N-3 fatty acids and the metabolic syndrome. Am J Clin Nutr 2006;83(Suppl):1499S–504S.

67. Rudkowska I. Fish oil for cardiovascular disease: impact on diabetes. Maturitas 2010;67:25–8.

68. Derweesh IH, Diblasio CJ, Kincade MC, et al. Risk of new-onset diabetes mellitus and worsening glycae-mic variables for established diabetes in men under-going androgen-deprivation therapy for prostate cancer. BJU Int 2007;100:1060–5.

69. Kris-Etherton PM, Harris WS, Appel LJ, et al. Omega-3 fatty acids and cardiovascular disease: new recom-mendations from the American Heart Association. Arterioscler Thromb Vasc Biol 2003;23:151–2.

70. Yokoyama M, Origasa H, Matsuzaki M, et al. Effects of eicosapentaenoic acid on major coronary events in

hypercholesterolaemic patients (JELIS): a randomized open-label, blinded endpoint analysis. Lancet 2007;369:1090–8.

71. Oikawa S, Yokoyama M, Origasa H, et al. Suppressive effect of EPA on the incidence of coronary events in hypercholesterolemia with impaired glucose metabolism: sub-analysis of the Japan EPA Lipid Intervention Study (JELIS). Atherosclerosis 2009;206:535–9.

72. Segal RJ, Reid RD, Coumeya KS, et al. Randomized controlled trial of resistance or aerobic exercise in men receiving radiation therapy for prostate cancer. J Clin Oncol 2009;27:344–51.

73. Barton DL, Soori GS, Bauer BA, et al. Pilot study of Panax quinquefolius (American ginseng) to improve cancer-related fatigue: a randomized, double-blind, dose-finding evaluation: NCCTG trial N03CA. Support Care Cancer 2010;18:179–87.

74. Kontos M, Agbaje OF, Rymer J, et al. What can be done about hot flushes after treatment for breast cancer? Climacteric 2010;13:4–21.

75. Moyad MA. Complementary therapies for reducing the risk of osteoporosis in patients receiving luteinizing hormone-releasing hormone treatment/orchiectomy for prostate cancer: a review and assessment of the need for more research. Urology 2002; 59(4 Suppl 1):34–40.

76. Irani J, Salomon L, Oba R, et al. Efficacy of venlafaxine, medroxyprogesterone acetate, and cyproterone acetate for the treatment of vasomotor hot flushes in men taking gonadotropin-releasing hormone analogues for prostate cancer: a double-blind, randomized trial. Lancet 2010;11:147–54.

77. Langenstroer P, Kramer B, Cutting B, et al. Parenteral medroxyprogesterone for the management of luteinizing hormone releasing hormone induced hot flashes in men with advanced prostate cancer. J Urol 2005;174:642–5.

78. Sullivan DH, Roberson PK, Smith ES, et al. Effects of muscle strength training and megestrol acetate on strength, muscle mass, and function in frail older people. J Am Geriatr Soc 2007;55:20–8.

79. Lambert CP, Sullivan DH, Evans WJ. Megesterol acetate-induced weight gain does not negatively affect blood lipids in elderly men: effects of resistance training and testosterone replacement. J Gerontol A Biol Sci Med Sci 2003;58:644–7.

80. Lucas M, Asselin G, Merette C, et al. Effects of ethyl-eicosapentaenoic acid omega-3 fatty acid supplementation on hot flashes and quality of life among middle-aged women: a double-blind, placebo-controlled, randomized clinical trial. Menopause 2009; 16:357–66.

81. Freeman MP. Omega-3 fatty acids in major depressive disorder. J Clin Psychiatry 2009;70(Suppl 5): 7–11.

82. Martins JG. EPA but not DHA appears to be responsible for the efficacy of omega-3 long chain polyunsaturated fatty acid supplementation in depression: evidence from a meta-analysis of randomized controlled trials. J Am Coll Nutr 2009; 28:525–42.

83. Wong RW, Rabie B. Chinese red yeast rice (Monascus purpureus-fermented rice) promotes bone formation. Chin Med 2008;3:4.

84. Majima T, Komatsu Y, Fukao A, et al. Short-term effects of atorvastatin on bone turnover in male patients with hypercholesterolemia. Endocr J 2007; 54:145–51.

85. Martin-Bautista E, Munoz-Torres M, Fonolla J, et al. Improvement of bone formation biomarkers after 1-year consumption with milk fortified with eicosapentaenoic acid, docosahexaenoic acid, oleic acid, and selected vitamins. Nutr Res 2010;30:320–6.

86. Murphy RA, Mourtzakis M, Chu QS, et al. Nutritional intervention with fish oil provides a benefit over standard of care for weight and skeletal muscle mass in patients with nonsmall cell lung cancer receiving chemotherapy. Cancer 2011;117:1775–82.

87. Murphy RA, Mourtzakis M, Chu QS, et al. Supplementation with fish oil increases first-line chemotherapy efficacy in patients with advanced nonsmall cell lung cancer. Cancer 2011. DOI:10.1002/cncr.25933. [Epub ahead of print].

88. Layman DK, Evans EM, Erickson D, et al. A moderate-protein diet produces sustained weight loss and long-term changes in body composition and blood lipids in obese adults. J Nutr 2009;139:514–21.

89. Dhillon PK, Kenfield SA, Stampfer MJ, et al. Long-term aspirin use and the risk of total, high-grade, regionally advanced and lethal prostate cancer in a prospective cohort of health professionals, 1988–2006. Int J Cancer 2011;128:2444–52.

90. Rothwell PM, Fowkes FG, Belch JF, et al. Effect of daily aspirin on long-term risk of death due to cancer: analysis of individual patient data from randomized trials. Lancet 2011;377:31–41.

91. Antithrombotic Trialists' (ATT) Collaboration. Aspirin in the primary and secondary prevention of vascular disease: collaborative meta-analysis of individual participant data from randomized trials. Lancet 2009;373:1849–60.

Lifestyle Recommendations to Reduce the Risk of Kidney Stones

Tiziana Meschi, MD, Antonio Nouvenne, MD, PhD, Loris Borghi, MD*

KEYWORDS

- Idiopathic calcium nephrolithiasis • Lifestyle • Diet
- Prevention • Kidney stones

Kidney stones are a disorder that could be termed social because of its vast diffusion and growing incidence in wealthy industrialized countries.[1] Many international studies have shown that this condition affects just less than 10% of the population, constituting an expense of approximately 2 billion dollars a year in hospital admissions in the United States alone.[2] In some cases, it is the consequence of specific hereditary or acquired diseases, such as cystinuria, primary hyperoxaluria, medullary sponge kidney, primary hyperparathyroidism, and infections or anatomic malformations of the kidneys and urinary tract. However, the most common form is idiopathic calcium nephrolithiasis (ICN), with the formation of calcium oxalate stones, sometimes mixed with calcium phosphate and with a prevalence of approximately 80%. The distribution by sex shows the frequency to be slightly higher in men.[3] The pathogenesis of ICN includes genetic and acquired factors that interact to cause biochemical urinary abnormalities that lead to the formation of kidney stones. A high rate of supersaturations of calcium oxalate and/or calcium phosphate leads to the formation of crystalline nests that can grow and join together to form a stone. The urinary elements and compounds, both inhibitors and activators, involved in the crystallization process are known as lithogenic urinary risk factors. For calcium oxalate, the lithogenic urinary risk factors are low urinary volume (<2 L/d), hypercalciuria (>250 mg/d), hyperoxaluria (>40 mg/d), hyperuricosuria (>600 mg/d), hypocitraturia (<320 mg/d), and hypomagnesuria (<50 mg/d). For calcium phosphate, in addition to the above, the most important factors are hyperphosphaturia (>1000 mg/d) and urinary pH. A pH more than 7 favors the formation of kidney stones primarily comprising phosphates, whereas a pH between 6 and 7 associated with a urinary volume of less than 1 L/d can dangerously increase the supersaturation of calcium phosphate and lead to the formation of mixed Ca-oxalate and Ca-phosphate stones. Last, in the case of uric acid–induced stone disease, another common form with a frequency of 10% to 15%, the factors involved are hyperuricosuria and pH less than 5.5. Of the various lithogenic urinary risk factors, the most commonly observed in patients with ICN is hypercalciuria, with a prevalence of approximately 50%. Regarding the age of onset, there are 2 peaks: between 20 and 30 years and between 50 and 60 years.[4]

The presence of a genetic substrate does not, however, detract from the role of lifestyle: dietary habits and lifestyle have a direct effect on the lithogenic urinary risk factors and the pathogenesis of this condition. This article examines the role of

This work was supported by Fondazione per la Ricerca Scientifica Termale (FoRST) grants.
The authors have nothing to disclose.
Internal Medicine and Subacute Critical Care Clinic, Department of Clinical Sciences, University of Parma, Via A. Gramsci 14, 43126 Parma, Italy
* Corresponding author.
E-mail address: loris.borghi@unipr.it

Urol Clin N Am 38 (2011) 313–320
doi:10.1016/j.ucl.2011.04.002

lifestyle in the prevention and treatment of calcium and uric acid kidney stones. This article specifically analyzes the relationship between (1) kidney stones and dietary habits, (2) kidney stones and body weight, (3) kidney stones and exercise, (4) kidney stones and stressful life events, and (5) particular causes.

KIDNEY STONES AND DIETARY HABITS

For many years now, diet has been known to play a key role in the development of kidney stones. Some authors postulate that the changes in the Western-style diet in recent decades have contributed substantially in increasing the prevalence of this condition. As this article shows, the foundations of an antilithogenic diet are correct intake of water, protein, salt, fruits and vegetables, milk and dairy products, carbohydrates, fats, and vitamins.

The Role of Water

The Equil program[5] makes it possible to simulate the changes in relative saturation of calcium oxalate, calcium phosphate, and uric acid when the urinary volume is increased from 0.5 to 3.0 L/d, keeping constant all the other urinary parameters involved in the calculation of the saturation point (**Fig. 1**). Such a urine composition reflects that seen in a healthy subject on a Western-style diet. With diuresis less than 1 L/d, even the urine of a normal subject reaches extremely high supersaturation levels, certainly high enough to promote

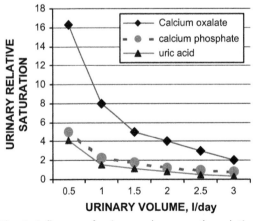

Fig. 1. Influence of urinary volume on the relative saturation for calcium oxalate, calcium phosphate, and uric acid. Simulations are made with the Equil program. Except volume, the other urinary parameters (pH, sodium, potassium, calcium, magnesium, ammonium, phosphorous, sulfate, oxalate, citrate, and uric acid) are kept constant. A value above 1 indicates supersaturation.

spontaneous crystallization of the lithogenic salts. If, on the other hand, the volume is kept more than 2.5 L/d, the urine becomes undersaturated for calcium phosphate and uric acid (<1) and only slightly supersaturated for calcium oxalate, making spontaneous crystallization impossible.[6] Given that, in the context of these physiologic variations in diuresis, ion excretion is largely independent of the urinary volume, this example simulates very closely what actually happens when water intake is high.[7] Moreover, the increase in diuretic volume does not affect the activity of the antilithogenic inhibitor molecules; in fact, the aggregation capacity of the crystals after an oxalate load is far lower in dilute urine than in concentrated urine.[8,9] Although for many years the only advice given to patients with kidney stones was to increase their water intake, there is only 1 randomized controlled study focusing on this practice, and it showed a significant reduction in the relapse rate and an increase in the time to relapse in patients whose urinary volume was constantly more than 2 L/d.[10,11]

However, large epidemiologic studies have indicated high urinary volume as an efficacious means of prevention in the general population, reducing the risk by 29% to 39%.[12–14]

An increase in fluids is, therefore, efficacious because it (1) reduces the urinary concentration of calcium, oxalate, and uric acid with a consequent reduction in the supersaturation of calcium oxalate, calcium phosphate, and uric acid; (2) increases the urinary tolerance to the oxalate load; (3) reduces the urinary concentration of macromolecules without altering their inhibitory power; and (4) increases the clearance of crystals and post–extracorporeal shockwave lithotripsy fragments.

The Role of Other Beverages

Whereas the role of water is now widely accepted, the role of other beverages is still controversial in literature. Most studies evaluated a surrogate end point (ie, lithogenic urinary risk factors), and there are little data available on studies with a long follow-up evaluating the effect on the onset or relapse of kidney stones.[15]

Beverages that exert a positive effect by raising pH, citrate, and/or urinary volume are available on the market (eg, freshly squeezed/industrially produced orange or lemon juice, coffee, green tea, beer, and wine). Blueberry juice is particularly useful in the treatment of infected stone disease, partly, because of its acidifying capacity.[16]

Other beverages increase oxalate (eg, tea) or are prolithogenic because of the mechanisms that are yet unclear (such as grapefruit and apple juice, and cola). In connection with this, because of the amount and frequency of consumption, soft drinks deserve a mention: recent studies have identified an increased risk of calcium- and uric acid–related stone disease because of soft drink consumption, probably because of their fructose, sucrose, and phosphoric acid contents.[17–20]

The sport and energy drinks, whose consumption in the Western countries is rising, constitute a category a part. The literature provides few and often contradictory studies evaluating the lithogenic urinary risk factors[21,22]: the energy/sport drinks rich in sodium, carbohydrates, and caffeine could increase the risk of kidney stones. However, further studies are required.

The Role of Proteins

The results of large epidemiologic studies are contradictory: whereas in a large cohort study of healthy men, a protein intake of more than 75 g/d led to a 33% increase in risk,[12] in the Nurses' Health Study (NHS) II study conducted on approximately 100,000 healthy women, an intake of more than 78 g led to a 16% reduction in risk. However, animal proteins have a different effect compared with that of plant proteins, and the prevalence of kidney stones among vegetarians is half that among the general population.[23] Two randomized controlled trials have studied the effects of a low-protein diet with a long follow-up. The first[24] studied, for 4 years, 99 patients at high risk for kidney stones randomized to receive either mineral water therapy alone or a low-protein, high-fiber diet. Recurrence was greater in the latter group than among controls. However, this study presents many biases, including a higher water intake in the control group, poor compliance with the low-protein diet, and differences in the calcium and fiber intakes between the 2 groups. The second study, conducted by the research group of this article,[25] followed up 120 patients, for 5 years, randomized to receive either a low-calcium diet or a low-protein, low-salt, and normal-calcium diet. In the latter group, the relapse rate was significantly lower (40% vs 20%). However, for this study, it was not possible to distinguish the protective effect of the reduction in protein from the increase in calcium and the reduction in sodium.

But why is it useful to limit animal proteins in any case? A diet containing too much protein can cause (1) hypercalciuria because of an increase in intestinal absorption of calcium, an increase in bone reabsorption, and a reduction in tubular calcium reabsorption; (2) hyperoxaluria because of an increase in intestinal absorption and in the endogenous production of oxalate; (3) hyperuricosuria

because of an increase in the intake and endogenous production of purines; and (d) hypocitraturia and reduction in pH caused by an increase in the fixed acid load.

The Role of Salt

Because of the difficulties in quantifying salt in diet questionnaires, the data available in the literature are contradictory. There is a direct relationship between calciuria and sodiuria (**Fig. 2**), and data exist[26] that a 2-g increase in dietary salt causes a 40-mg (1 mmol) increase in calciuria in healthy subjects and an 80-mg (2 mmol) increase in calciuria in patients with hypercalciuric kidney stones. It also has a cumulative effect with proteins.

The authors also recently demonstrated that a moderately low-salt diet is able to correct hypercalciuria in subjects with calcium stone disease with hypercalciuria.[27] Moreover, the same reduction in salt normalizes urinary oxalate values in patients with mild hyperoxaluria.[28]

So why salt must be reduced? Too much salt can lead to (1) hypercalciuria because of a reduction in the tubular reabsorption of calcium both with a direct mechanism and as a consequence of the expansion in the extracellular volume, the mobilization of bone calcium, and an increase in the intestinal reabsorption; and (2) hypocitraturia because of cellular potassium deficiency and an increase in acid load.[29,30]

The Role of Fruits and Vegetables

Fruits and vegetables can have an antilithogenic effect. Their beneficial effects are related to the specific chemical/physical and nutritional characteristics of these foods, which have a high water, potassium, and magnesium content; a low sodium chloride content; and a high alkalinization power because of the presence of bicarbonate and citrate. A high potassium and magnesium intake reduces the risk of kidney stones by up to 50%.[13,14]

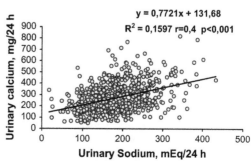

Fig. 2. Relationship between urinary sodium and calcium in 743 men normotensive with ICN.

In 2004, the authors demonstrated that deprivation of fruits and vegetables can cause a significant reduction in citraturia and an increase in calciuria even in healthy subjects, whereas, conversely, supplementation of fruits and vegetables in patients at high risk for hypocitraturic stone disease corrects the deficiency.[31] Recently, 2 large cohort studies confirmed this experimental evidence.[32,33] Taylor and colleagues assessed the diets of approximately 240,000 subjects participating in 3 large cohort studies: Health Professionals Follow-Up Study, NHS I, and NHS II.

These authors defined a Dietary Approaches to Stop Hypertension (DASH) score based on 8 components: a high intake of fruits, vegetables, nuts and legumes, low-fat dairy products, and whole grains and a low intake of sodium, sweetened beverages, and red and processed meats. Over a combined 50 years' follow-up, they documented that higher DASH scores were associated with a marked decrease in the risk of kidney stones.

In a recent study conducted in 2010, Taylor and colleagues[33] found that a DASH-style diet was associated with an increased urinary output, regardless of the fluid intake. They speculated that higher urinary volumes were a result of the higher food water content and reported that a high dietary intake of fruits and vegetables was linked to increased urinary citrate levels and higher urinary pH.

So why is it useful to increase the consumption of fruits and vegetables? A deficiency of alkaline potassium, magnesium, and fiber in the diet can cause (1) hypercalciuria because of a reduction in the tubular reabsorption of calcium, excess free intestinal calcium, and mobilization of bone calcium; (2) hypocitraturia because of the depletion of intracellular potassium with consequent mild intracellular acidosis; and (3) promotion of the tendency to crystallization of calcium oxalate caused by a deficiency in magnesium with consequent hypomagnesuria.

The Role of Milk and Dairy Products

Calcium intake is known to cause an 8% increase in calciuria in controls and a 20% increase in subjects prone to kidney stones.[34] However, a restriction in dietary calcium is not advisable in patients at high risk for kidney stones. Indeed, in a large number of subjects, a low-calcium diet does not reduce calciuria, and by reducing the calcium intake, it increases the intestinal absorption of oxalate and hence oxaluria. Last, very often, the imposed reduction of dairy products leads to an increase in the patients' protein intake.[35,36]

Curhan and colleagues, in the previously mentioned NHS II study, evaluated approximately 100,000 healthy women and reported a 35% reduction in risk when calcium intake exceeded 1098 mg/d.

In our study,[25] the relapse rate was significantly lower in patients on a normal-calcium, low-protein, low-salt diet than in patients on a low-calcium diet, both in subjects at high and low risk of relapse.

Dietary calcium deficiency can lead to a reduction in calciuria because of lower intestinal absorption but also an increase in calciuria because of a loss in calcium from the bone. Last, the reduced concentration of calcium in the distal intestine causes an increase in free oxalate because of absorption and hence hyperoxaluria.

The Role of Carbohydrates, Fats, and Vitamins

It is well known that glucose load causes a rise in urinary calcium level and the entity of this effect is greater in patients at high risk for kidney stones and their families than in controls.[37]

A simple intake of sugar is associated with an increase in the risk of stone disease in women but not in men. Insulin may affect the tubular reabsorption of calcium. Insulin resistance, metabolic syndrome, and type 2 diabetes have been associated with kidney stones, particularly those caused by uric acid. Indeed, insulin resistance can interfere with the renal production of ammonia and cause a decrease in pH, with a concomitant reduction in citrate and precipitation of uric acid crystals. Moreover, optimal glycemic control in patients with diabetes leads to a significant reduction in calciuria.

It has also been suggested that a relationship exists between fats and kidney stones: a high-fat, high-cholesterol diet can cause stone disease in rats, and fat intake correlates with oxalate excretion. In contrast, a good intake of fish oil, a source of omega-3 fatty acids, reduces not merely calciuria and oxaluria but also certain proinflammatory cytokines.[38–41]

The vitamins thought to be involved in the lithogenic risk are vitamins D, C, B6, and A. Certain subjects with idiopathic hypercalciuria have excess vitamin D in their blood with an increase in the intestinal absorption of calcium. However, epidemiologic studies with long follow-ups did not show any association between vitamin D intake and the lithogenic risk; indeed in the industrialized countries, a vitamin D deficiency is more likely because of the little time spent outdoors.[42,43]

Over the past decade, vitamin C supplementation has become a common practice in the Western countries. Ascorbic acid is an oxalate precursor, and therefore, an excessive intake is to be discouraged in subjects with kidney stones (a maximum dosage of 1500 mg/d is recommended).

Vitamin B6 is involved in oxalic acid metabolism, and a deficiency causes an increase in the endogenous production of oxalate. Use of vitamin B6 supplement can be considered to treat hyperoxaluria.[44,45]

Vitamin A is an antioxidant and reduces the cell damage caused by crystal deposition. In animal trials but not on humans, vitamin A supplementation reduces the lithogenic risk and increases citraturia, despite that its mechanism is unknown.[46]

KIDNEY STONES AND BODY WEIGHT

The role of body weight, body mass index (BMI), and body composition in determining the lithogenic risk remains a subject for debate. Large epidemiologic studies[47,48] have documented an increase in the risk of kidney stones with an increase in body weight, BMI, and waist circumference. However, this increase in risk is accompanied by a redistribution in the type of stone disease in the overweight population compared with the general population, with a decrease in the prevalence of calcium stone disease and an increase in the prevalence of uric acid stone disease.[49,50] The increase in lean mass was associated with an increase in the incidence for men alone.[51] Moreover, weight loss is not associated with a reduction in risk.[48]

Regarding the lithogenic urinary risk factors, an inverse relationship has been established between pH and BMI and between pH and fatty mass.[52] Furthermore, oxalate excretion has been related to body weight, body surface area, and lean mass.[53] An increase in BMI also boosts the excretion of oxalate, uric acid, sodium, phosphate, and calcium.[54–56] However, calcium does not remain significant if corrected for sodium and phosphate.[54]

Some recent retrospective studies[57–59] have described a positive relationship between the lithogenic urinary risk factors and excess weight and obesity. However, supersaturation values often do not change because the excretion of inhibitors and the intake of water also increase with an increase in weight and/or BMI percentiles. A common limitation to many of the studies quoted is that they did not evaluate dietary habits, in particular, protein intake. There is growing evidence that a high BMI and insulin resistance (ie, metabolic syndrome) are the etiologic factors of uric acid stone disease; because insulin stimulates the renal production of ammonium, insulin resistance may reduce the excretion of ammonium. Daudon and colleagues[60] demonstrated a 35.7% prevalence of uric acid stone disease in patients with type 2 diabetes compared with 11.3% in those without diabetes.

KIDNEY STONES AND EXERCISE

The effects of exercise on reducing the risk of stone disease and on the lithogenic urinary risk factors have been studied in very few studies and on a limited number of patients. On the other hand, there is a significant amount of evidence correlating immobility or bed rest with a high risk of stone disease. Many experimental models have been performed on astronauts in the absence of gravity. The 2 most important studies assessing moderate exercise (70%–75% VO_2max)[61,62] revealed an increase in the lithogenic urinary risk factors only in the absence of adequate hydration during and after exercise. Conversely, the results of many studies have shown exercise to have a beneficial effect on health and, therefore, hypothetically also on the risk of stone disease and related metabolic conditions. Indeed, exercise improves blood pressure control,[63] increases renal plasma flow,[64] reduces proinflammatory cytokines, and improves insulin sensitivity.[65]

KIDNEY STONES AND STRESSFUL LIFE EVENTS

A stressful lifestyle is associated with a higher risk of stone disease. This has been proved particularly in women. Stress increases not only the risk of onset of the disease but also the frequency of passage of stones already present. The physiopathologic mechanism has not been entirely clarified, although it would seem that hormonal causes are involved, and stress reduces certain antilithogenic factors such as magnesium and citrate, whereas calciuria, oxaluria, and uricosuria increase in response to stressful events.[66]

PARTICULAR CAUSES
Melamine

In recent years, data have emerged about a possible relationship between environmental exposure to dietary additives and the development of kidney stones. In China, in late 2008, many cases (the estimated figure is 50,000) of kidney stones were observed in the pediatric population, whose spontaneous incidence is known to be very low. This epidemic was related to the consumption of powdered milk contaminated with melamine, a dietary additive used, legally, to increase the nitrogen content in certain types of animal feed. When added to human food products, it can falsify their protein content and is, therefore, considered a sophistication.[67]

Melamine, which usually forms salts with cyanuric acid, precipitates in the distal renal tubule, constituting the matrix for the formation of stones, which are usually found in the renal pelvis and have irregular dimensions that are not easily seen on ultrasonographic images.

Because the toxicity of melamine in humans was unknown until 2008, further studies are needed; however, it cannot be ruled out that exposure to this toxic agent can increase the risk of kidney stone disease also in adults, and similarly, the long-term effects of even episodic exposure are not yet known. In addition, the enormous amount of food additives that humans are exposed every day can, in some way, influence the risk of kidney stones, but evidence is lacking on this topic.[67]

Betel Quid Chewers

The chewing of betel quid is a common practice in many countries, particularly in Southeast Asia. The quid is a preparation of betel leaf, areca nut, and chuna (ie, calcium hydroxide paste). Betel quid chewers suffer from hypercalciuria, alkaline urine, and hypocitraturia, with the risk of developing calcium phosphate and calcium oxalate stones. The presence of calcium hydroxide chuna would seem to be the main cause that, also, exposes subjects to a greater risk of developing milk-alkali syndrome.[68]

Box 1
Ten rules for the prevention of the risk of kidney stones

1. Keep an ideal weight and take regular moderate exercise in the open air.
2. Drink enough water to obtain a urinary volume of 2 L/d.
3. Restrict the intake of meat and poultry proteins to about 20 g/d.
4. Eat about 40 g of plant protein a day.
5. Eat fruits and vegetables every day, avoiding products rich in oxalate.
6. Eat milk and dairy products to achieve a calcium intake of about 1000 mg/d.
7. Follow the international guidelines on fat and carbohydrate consumption.
8. Use fresh and frozen food products, avoiding precooked and/or preserved foods.
9. Avoid do-it-yourself use of supplements and only take medicines and supplements under medical supervision.
10. Try to avoid stressful life events as far as possible.

Ephedrine

Ephedrine and its metabolites are alkaloids extracted from plants of the *Ephedra* species and have alpha- and beta-adrenergic activities. In the official pharmacopoeia, they are used as nasal decongestants for topical use. However, many natural herbal remedies favoring weight loss and improving physical and mental performance contain varying quantities of these alkaloids. The sometimes severe and potentially lethal side effects of these preparations include precipitation in the renal tubules with the formation of radiolucent stones, and the prevalence of this form of stone disease in the United States is 0.06%.[69]

SUMMARY

Diet and lifestyle choices have a significant influence on the risk of kidney stones. Both doctors and patients should be educated to consider a healthy lifestyle as an efficacious medical approach. **Box 1** shows a simple list of 10 rules for the prevention of the risk of kidney stones. It would be useful to have evidence from controlled studies evaluating the long-term effects of diet and lifestyle modifications compared with medical therapy and clarifying the relationships between kidney stones, weight, and body mass.

REFERENCES

1. Goldfarb DS. Increasing prevalence of kidney stones in the United States. Kidney Int 2003;63: 1951–2.
2. Clark JY, Thompson IM, Optenberg SA. Economic impact of urolithiasis in the United States. J Urol 1995;154:2020–4.
3. Soucie JM, Thun MJ, Coates RJ, et al. Demographic and geographic variability of kidney stones in the United States. Kidney Int 1994;46:893–9.
4. Worcester EM, Coe FL. Clinical practice. Calcium kidney stones. N Engl J Med 2010;363:954–63.
5. Werness PG, Brown CM, Smith LH, et al. Equil 2: a basic computer program for the calculation of urinary saturation. J Urol 1985;134:1242–4.
6. Pak CY, Sakhaee K, Crowther C, et al. Evidence justifying a high fluid intake in treatment of nephrolithiasis. Ann Intern Med 1980;93:36–9.
7. Borghi L, Guerra A, Meschi T, et al. Relationship between supersaturation and calcium oxalate crystallization in normals and idiopathic calcium oxalate stone formers. Kidney Int 1999;55:1041–50.
8. Guerra A, Meschi T, Allegri F, et al. Concentrated urine and diluted urine: the effects of citrate and magnesium on the crystallization of calcium oxalate induced in vitro by an oxalate load. Urol Res 2006; 34:359–64.

9. Guerra A, Allegri F, Meschi T, et al. Effects of urine dilution on quantity, size and aggregation of calcium oxalate crystals induced in vitro by an oxalate load. Clin Chem Lab Med 2005;43:585–9.

10. Borghi L, Meschi T, Amato F, et al. Urinary volume, water and recurrences in idiopathic calcium nephrolithiasis: a 5-year randomized prospective study. J Urol 1996;155:839–43.

11. Qiang W, Ke Z. Water for preventing urinary calculi. Cochrane Database Syst Rev 2004;3:CD004292.

12. Curhan GC, Willet WC, Rimm EB, et al. A prospective study of dietary calcium and other nutrients and the risk of symptomatic kidney stones. N Engl J Med 1993;328:833–8.

13. Curhan GC, Willett WC, Knight EL, et al. Dietary factors and the risk of incident kidney stones in younger women. Arch Intern Med 2004;164:885–91.

14. Taylor EN, Stampfer MJ, Curhan GC. Dietary factors and the risk of incident kidney stones in men: new insights after 14 years of follow-up. J Am Soc Nephrol 2004;15:3225–32.

15. Curhan GC, Willett WC, Speizer FE, et al. Beverage use and risk for kidney stones in women. Ann Intern Med 1998;128:534–40.

16. Taylor EN, Curhan GC. Determinants of 24-hour urinary oxalate excretion. Clin J Am Soc Nephrol 2008;3:1453–60.

17. Taylor EN, Curhan GC. Fructose consumption and the risk of kidney stones. Kidney Int 2008;73:207–12.

18. Asselman M, Verkoelen CF. Fructose intake as a risk factor for kidney stone disease. Kidney Int 2008;73:139–40.

19. Choi HK, Curhan G. Soft drinks, fructose consumption, and the risk of gout in men: prospective cohort study. BMJ 2008;336:309–12.

20. Choi HK, Willett W, Curhan G. Fructose-rich beverages and risk of gout in women. JAMA 2010;304:2270–8.

21. Passman CM, Holmes RP, Knight J, et al. Effect of soda consumption on urinary stone risk parameters. J Endourol 2009;23:347–50.

22. Goodman JW, Asplin JR, Goldfarb DS. Effect of two sports drinks on urinary lithogenicity. Urol Res 2009;37:41–6.

23. Robertson WG, Peacock M, Marshall DH. Prevalence of urinary stone disease in vegetarians. Eur Urol 1982;8:334–9.

24. Hiatt RA, Ettinger B, Caan B, et al. Randomized controlled trial of a low animal protein, high fiber diet in the prevention of recurrent calcium oxalate kidney stones. Am J Epidemiol 1996;144:25–33.

25. Borghi L, Schianchi T, Meschi T, et al. Comparison of two diets for the prevention of recurrent stones in idiopathic hypercalciuria. N Engl J Med 2002;346:77–84.

26. Massey LK, Whiting SJ. Dietary salt, urinary calcium, and kidney stone risk. Nutr Rev 1995;53:131–4.

27. Nouvenne A, Meschi T, Prati B, et al. Effects of a low-salt diet on idiopathic hypercalciuria in calcium-oxalate stone formers: a 3-mo randomized controlled trial. Am J Clin Nutr 2010;91:565–70.

28. Nouvenne A, Meschi T, Guerra A, et al. Diet to reduce mild hyperoxaluria in patients with idiopathic calcium oxalate stone formation: a pilot study. Urology 2009;73:725–30.

29. Kok DJ, Iestra JA, Doorenbos CJ, et al. The effects of dietary excesses in animal protein and in sodium on the composition and the crystallization kinetics of calcium oxalate monohydrate in urines of healthy men. J Clin Endocrinol Metab 1990;71:861–7.

30. Dahl LK. Possible role of salt intake in the development of essential hypertension. Int J Epidemiol 2005;34:967–78.

31. Meschi T, Maggiore U, Fiaccadori E, et al. The effect of fruits and vegetables on urinary stone risk factors. Kidney Int 2004;66:2402–10.

32. Taylor EN, Fung TT, Curhan GC. DASH-style diet associates with reduced risk for kidney stones. J Am Soc Nephrol 2009;20:2253–9.

33. Taylor EN, Stampfer MJ, Mount DB, et al. DASH-style diet and 24-hour urine composition. Clin J Am Soc Nephrol 2010;5:2315–22.

34. Coe FL, Favus MJ, Crockett T, et al. Effects of low-calcium diet on urine calcium excretion, parathyroid function and serum 1,25 (OH)2D3 levels in patients with idiopathic hypercalciuria and in normal subjects. Am J Med 1982;72:25–32.

35. Lemann J Jr, Adams ND, Gray RW. Urinary calcium excretion in human beings. N Engl J Med 1979;30:535–41.

36. Martini LA, Heilberg IP. Stop dietary calcium restriction in kidney stone-forming patients. Nutr Rev 2002;60:212–4.

37. Lemann J Jr, Piering WF, Lennon E. Possible role of carbohydrate-induced calciuria in calcium oxalate kidney-stone formation. N Engl J Med 1969;280:232–7.

38. Baggio B, Budakovic A, Nassuato MA, et al. Plasma phospholipid arachidonic acid content and calcium metabolism in idiopathic calcium nephrolithiasis. Kidney Int 2000;58:1278–84.

39. Baggio B, Gambero G, Zambon S, et al. Anomalous phospholipid n-6 polyunsaturated fatty acid composition in idiopathic calcium nephrolithiasis. J Am Soc Nephrol 1996;7:613–20.

40. Buck AC, Davies R, Harrison T. The protective role of eicosapentaenoic acid (EPA) in the pathogenesis of nephrolithiasis. J Urol 1991;146:188–94.

41. Taylor EN, Stampfer MJ, Curhan GC. Fatty acid intake and incident nephrolithiasis. Am J Kidney Dis 2005;45:267–74.

42. Curhan GC, Willett WC, Rimm EB, et al. A prospective study of the intake of vitamins C and B6,

and the risk of kidney stones in men. J Urol 1996; 155:1847–51.

43. Curhan GC, Willett WC, Speizer FE, et al. Intake of vitamins B6 and C and the risk of kidney stones in women. J Am Soc Nephrol 1999;10:840–5.

44. Di Tommaso L, Tolomelli B, Mezzini R, et al. Renal calcium phosphate and oxalate deposition in prolonged vitamin B6 deficiency: studies on a rat model of urolithiasis. BJU Int 2002;89:571–5.

45. Chetyrkin SV, Kim D, Belmont JM, et al. Pyridoxamine lowers kidney crystals in experimental hyperoxaluria: a potential therapy for primary hyperoxaluria. Kidney Int 2005;67:56–60.

46. Bardaoui M, Sakly R, Neffati F, et al. Effect of vitamin A supplemented diet on calcium oxalate renal stone formation in rats. Exp Toxicol Pathol 2010;62:573–6.

47. Curhan GC, Willett WC, Rimm EB, et al. Body size and risk of kidney stones. J Am Soc Nephrol 1998; 9:1645–52.

48. Taylor EN, Stampfer MJ, Curhan GC. Obesity, weight gain, and the risk of kidney stones. JAMA 2005; 293(4):455–62.

49. Lee SC, Kim YJ, Kim TH, et al. Impact of obesity in patients with urolithiasis and its prognostic usefulness in stone recurrence. J Urol 2008;179:570–4.

50. Ekeruo WO, Tan YH, Young MD, et al. Metabolic risk factors and the impact of medical therapy on the management of nephrolithiasis in obese patients. J Urol 2004;172:159–63.

51. Curhan GC, Willett WC, Speizer FE, et al. Twenty-four-hour urine chemistries and the risk of kidney stones among women and men. Kidney Int 2001; 59:2290–8.

52. Remer T, Berkemeyer S, Rylander R, et al. Muscularity and adiposity in addition to net acid excretion as predictors of 24-hour urinary pH in young adults and elderly. Eur J Clin Nutr 2007;61:605–9.

53. Lemann J Jr, Pleuss JA, Worcester EM, et al. Urinary oxalate excretion increases with body size and decreases with increasing dietary calcium intake among healthy adults. Kidney Int 1996;49: 200–8.

54. Taylor EN, Curhan GC. Body size and 24-hour urine composition. Am J Kidney Dis 2006;48(6): 905–15.

55. Siener R, Glatz S, Nicolay C, et al. The role of overweight and obesity in calcium oxalate stone formation. Obes Res 2004;12:106–13.

56. Duffey BG, Pedro RN, Kriedberg C, et al. Lithogenic risk factors in the morbidly obese population. J Urol 2008;179:1401–6.

57. Eisner BH, Eisenberg ML, Stoller ML. Relationship between body mass index and quantitative 24-hour urine chemistries in patients with nephrolithiasis. Urology 2010;75:1289–93.

58. Negri AL, Spivacow FR, Del Valle EE, et al. Role of overweight and obesity on the urinary excretion of promoters and inhibitors of stone formation in stone formers. Urol Res 2008;36:303–7.

59. Sarica K, Altay B, Erturhan S. Effect of being overweight on stone-forming risk factors. Urology 2008; 71:771–5.

60. Daudon M, Traxer O, Conort P, et al. Type 2 diabetes increases the risk for uric acid stones. J Am Soc Nephrol 2006;17:2026–33.

61. Sakhaee K, Nigam S, Snell P, et al. Assessment of the pathogenetic role of physical exercise in renal stone formation. J Clin Endocrinol Metab 1987;65:974–9.

62. Sriboonlue P, Prasongwatana V, Tosukhowong P, et al. Increased risk of urinary stone disease by physical exercise. Southeast Asian J Trop Med Public Health 1996;27:172–7.

63. Lin JS, O'Connor E, Whitlock EP, et al. Behavioral counseling to promote physical activity and a healthful diet to prevent cardiovascular disease in adults: a systematic review for the U.S. Preventive Services Task Force. Ann Intern Med 2010;153:736–50.

64. McAllister RM. Adaptations in control of blood flow with training: splanchnic and renal blood flows. Med Sci Sports Exerc 1998;30:375–81.

65. Hansen D, Dendale P, van Loon LJ, et al. The impact of training modalities on the clinical benefits of exercise intervention in patients with cardiovascular disease risk or type 2 diabetes mellitus. Sports Med 2010;40:921–40.

66. Najem GR, Seebode JJ, Samady AJ, et al. Stressful life events and risk of symptomatic kidney stones. Int J Epidemiol 1997;26:1017–23.

67. Bhalla V, Grimm PC, Chertow GM, et al. Melamine nephrotoxicity: an emerging epidemic in an era of globalization. Kidney Int 2009;75:774–9.

68. Allen SE, Singh S, Robertson WG. The increased risk of urinary stone disease in betel quid chewers. Urol Res 2006;34:239–43.

69. Powell T, Hsu FF, Turk J, et al. Ma-huang strikes again: ephedrine nephrolithiasis. Am J Kidney Dis 1998;32:153–9.

Molecular Markers that Can Be Utilized in Diet and Dietary Supplement Research

Mark A. Moyad, MD, MPH[a,b,*], Kirk J. Wojno, MD[c]

KEYWORDS

- Diet • Diet supplements • Molecular markers
- Urological cancer

So many markers and so little time and financing should be the new adage. Prostate and other cancers have a multitude of potential markers that can be used in studies, including those that test diet and dietary supplement interventions.[1–5] More overt clinical markers include imaging tests, biopsy results, and prostate-specific antigen kinetics. However, because it is not realistic to follow men in clinical trials for decades on nutritional interventions, researchers are relying on numerous molecular markers to access the potential impact of interventions on urological and other cancers. This article briefly reviews some of the diverse markers that may be considered by a researcher for use in a clinical study.

ANTIAPOPTOTIC PROTEINS

When affected favorably by diet and dietary supplements or another intervention, there should be a downregulation of antiapoptotic proteins,[6] because upregulation or overexpression of these proteins promotes cancer cell survival, resistance to conventional treatments, and progression. Examples of common antiapoptotic proteins used in studies include Bcl-2 (B-cell lymphoma 2),[7] Bcl-XL,[8,9] Bfl1/A1,[10] c-FLIP (cellular FLICE inhibitory pathway) that contains multiple apoptosis inhibitors,[11] cIAP (cellular inhibitor of apoptosis),[12] survivin,[13] TRAF1 (tumor necrosis factor receptor–associated factor),[14] and XIAP (X-linked inhibitor of apoptosis).[15]

APOPTOTIC PROTEINS

These proteins need to be upregulated or hyperactivated in diet and supplement studies, because potentially more apoptosis of unhealthy or malignant cells would occur if the intervention had a positive impact.[16] Examples of apoptotic proteins include Bax,[17] caspase (2, 3, 7, 9, and so forth),[18] and PARP (poly(ADP-ribose) polymerase 1).[19]

CELL ADHESION MOLECULES

Cell adhesion molecules (CAMs) and integrins are needed for the maintenance of the epithelium.[20–24] An abnormality or insult in epithelial cell adhesion can lead to invasive and metastatic behavior whereby cells invade the basement membrane and access the stroma. Loss of adhesion molecules is more characteristic of aggressiveness, but so is the overexpression of some of these molecules. Moreover, effective interventions appear to maintain or restore CAMs in some instances. Multiple CAMs exist, including ELAM (endothelial leukocyte adhesion molecule), ICAM-1 (intercellular cell adhesion molecule 1), VCAM (vascular cellular adhesion molecule), cadherins, and integrins.

a Department of Urology, University of Michigan Medical Center, 1500 East Medical Center Drive, Ann Arbor, MI 48109-0330, USA
b Eisenhower Wellness Institute, Eisenhower Medical Center, Rancho Mirage, CA, USA
c Comprehensive Medical Center, Pathology, Royal Oak, MI 48073, USA
* Corresponding author. Department of Urology, University of Michigan Medical Center, 1500 East Medical Center Drive, Ann Arbor, MI 48109-0330.
E-mail address: moyad@umich.edu

Urol Clin N Am 38 (2011) 321–324
doi:10.1016/j.ucl.2011.05.006
0094-0143/11/$ – see front matter © 2011 Elsevier Inc. All rights reserved.

CELL CYCLE PROTEINS

Cell cycle proteins are switches that allow the cell cycle or replication to continue, cease, or even discontinue.[25–27] An intervention that favorably affects the cell cycle is of enormous interest. Several commonly tested cell cycle proteins include CDK (cyclin-dependent kinase), cyclins, p21, p27, and p57.

GROWTH FACTORS/ANGIOGENESIS/ PROLIFERATION/INFLAMMATORY COMPOUNDS

Agents such as celecoxib that can downregulate growth factors or markers of inflammation may

have anticancer activity.[28,29] The potential benefits or lack of benefit of fish oil has been studied via COX-2 (cyclooxygenase-2), IL (interleukin)-6, and TNF-α (tumor necrosis factor α) pathways.[30–32]

Reductions or downregulation of growth factors appears to be a favorable sign for a diet or dietary intervention. Some examples of compounds in this category include COX-2,[33] EGF (epidermal growth factor),[34] erythropoietin and receptor,[35] Ki67,[36] FGF (fibroblast growth factor),[37,38] IGF (insulin-like growth factor),[39,40] IL-1, IL-6, IL-8,[41–43] PDGF (platelet-derived growth factor),[44] TGF-β (transforming growth factor β),[45] TNF-α,[46] and VEGF (vascular endothelial growth factor).[47]

MISCELLANEOUS

Protein kinases are enzymes that assist in modifying other proteins via phosphorylation and in some cases increasing aggressiveness. For example, upregulation of phosphorylated Akt may increase drug resistance,[48] and similar concerns occur with HER-2 expression.[49] Transcription factors such as NF-κB (nuclear factor κB) affect signaling that can lead to inflammation and cancer progression.[50]

SUMMARY

Urological cancers have a multitude of potential molecular markers that can be used in laboratory and clinical studies of diet and dietary supplement interventions (**Table 1**). The decision as to which markers to use is difficult, but enough multiple diet and dietary supplement studies have been conducted over the past decade to allow researchers to compare results. Antiapoptotic and apoptotic proteins, CAMs, cell cycle compounds, growth factors, angiogenic markers, and proliferative and inflammatory signals have all been used in the past. Protein kinases and transcription factors should also be considered to gain a more diverse perspective. Testing with numerous molecular markers has become critical in gaining preliminary insight into the potential impact of a novel diet and supplemental agents.

Table 1
Molecular markers that could be used in diet and dietary supplement studies and cancer

Marker for Study	Examples
I. Antiapoptotic proteins (downregulation suggests a beneficial impact by an intervention)	Bcl-2 Bcl-XL Bfl1/A1 c-FLIP cIAP Survivin TRAF1 XIAP
II. Apoptotic proteins (upregulation suggests a beneficial impact by an intervention)	Bax Caspase (2, 3, 7, 9, etc) PARP
III. Cell adhesion molecules (upregulation of some and downregulation of others suggests a beneficial impact by an intervention)	Cadherins ELAM ICAM-1 Integrins VCAM
IV. Cell cycle proteins (upregulation of some and downregulation of others suggests a beneficial impact by an intervention)	CDK Cyclins p21 p27 p57
V. Growth factors (down-regulation suggests a beneficial impact by an intervention)	COX-2 EGF Erythropoietin Ki67 FGF IGF IL-1, IL-6, IL-8 PDGF TGF-β TNF VEGF
VI. Miscellaneous (downregulation suggests a beneficial impact by an intervention, but there are exceptions)	Protein kinases (Akt, HER2) Transcription factors (NF-κB)

REFERENCES

1. Lippman SM, Klein EA, Goodman PJ, et al. Effect of selenium and vitamin E on risk of prostate cancer and other cancers: the Selenium and Vitamin E Cancer Prevention Trial (SELECT). JAMA 2009;301: 39–51.

2. Gaziano JM, Glynn RJ, Christen WG, et al. Vitamins E and C in the prevention of prostate and total cancer in men: the Physicians' Health Study II randomized controlled trial. JAMA 2009;301:52–62.

3. Zummerova A, Bohmer D, Fillo J, et al. The role of molecular biology in detection and monitoring of prostate cancer. Cesk Patol 2010;46:95–7.

4. Dunn BK, Jegalian K, Greenwald P. Biomarkers for early detection and as surrogate endpoints in cancer prevention trials: issues and opportunities. Recent Results Cancer Res 2011;188:21–47.

5. Ferte C, Andre F, Soria JC. Molecular circuits of solid tumors: prognostic and predictive tools for bedside use. Nat Rev Clin Oncol 2010;7:367–80.

6. Wilson TR, Johnston PG, Longley DB. Anti-apoptotic mechanisms of drug resistance in cancer. Curr Cancer Drug Targets 2009;9:307–19.

7. Hockenberry D, Zutter M, Hickey W, et al. Bcl-2 protein is an inner mitochondrial membrane protein that blocks topographically programmed cell death. Nature 1990;348:334–6.

8. Zhou F, Yang Y, Xing D. Bcl-2 and Bcl-xL play important roles in the crosstalk between autophagy and apoptosis. FEBS J 2011;278:403–13.

9. Datta R, Manome Y, Taneja N. Overexpression of Bcl-XL by cytotoxic drug exposure confers resistance to ionizing radiation-induced internucleosomal DNA fragmentation. Cell Growth Differ 1995;6:363–70.

10. Gimenez-Bonafe P, Tortosa A, Perez-Tomas R. Overcoming drug resistance by enhancing apoptosis of tumor cells. Curr Cancer Drug Targets 2009;9:320–40.

11. Bagnoli M, Canevari S, Mezzanzanica D. Cellular FLICE-inhibitory protein (C-FLIP) signaling: a key regulator of receptor-mediated apoptosis in physiologic context and in cancer. Int J Biochem Cell Biol 2010;42:210–3.

12. Gill C, Dowling C, O'Neill AJ, et al. Effects of cIAP-1, cIAP-2 and XIAP triple knockdown on prostate cancer cell susceptibility to apoptosis, cell survival and proliferation. Mol Cancer 2009;8:39.

13. Cheung CH, Cheng L, Chang KY, et al. Investigations of survivin: the past, present and future. Front Biosci 2011;16:952–61.

14. Arron JR, Walsh MC, Choi Y. TRAF-mediated TNFR-family signaling. Curr Protoc Immunol 2002;Chapter 11:Unit 11.9D.(Suppl 51):1–14.

15. Kashkar H. X-linked inhibitor of apoptosis: a chemoresistance factor or a hollow promise. Clin Cancer Res 2010;16:4496–502.

16. Shehzad A, Wahid F, Lee YS. Curcumin in cancer chemoprevention: molecular targets, pharmacokinetics, bioavailability, and clinical trials. Arch Pham (Weinheim) 2010;343:489–99.

17. Almubarak H, Jones A, Chaisuparat R, et al. Zoledronic acid directly suppresses cell proliferation and induces apoptosis in highly tumorigenic prostate and breast cancers. J Carcinog 2011;10:2.

18. Coffey RN, Watson RW, Fitzpatrick JM. Signaling for the caspases: their role in prostate cell apoptosis. J Urol 2001;165:5–14.

19. Dong Y, Bey EA, Li LS, et al. Prostate cancer radio-sensitization through poly(ADP-Ribose) polymerase-1 hyperactivation. Cancer Res 2010;70:8088–96.

20. Moschos SJ, Drogowski LM, Reppert SL, et al. Integrins and cancer. Oncology (Williston Oark) 2007;21(9 Suppl 3):13–20.

21. Angelucci C, Lama G, Lacopino F, et al. Leuprorelin acetate affects adhesion molecule expression in human prostate cancer cells. Int J Oncol 2011;38:1501–9.

22. Pontes-Junior J, Reis ST, Dall'Oglio M, et al. Evaluation of the expression of integrins and cell adhesion molecules through tissue microarray in lymph node metastases of prostate cancer. J Carcinog 2009;8:3.

23. Saha B, Arase A, Imam SS, et al. Overexpression of E-cadherin and beta-catenin proteins in metastatic prostate cancer cells in bone. Prostate 2008;68:78–84.

24. Desgrosellier JS, Cheresh DA. Integrins in cancer: biological implications and therapeutic opportunities. Nat Rev Cancer 2010;10:9–22.

25. Caldon CE, Sutherland RL, Musgrove E. Cell cycle proteins in epithelial differentiation: implications for breast cancer. Cell Cycle 2010;9:1918–28.

26. Rosenblatt R, Jonmarker S, Lewensohn R, et al. Current status of prognostic immunohistochemical markers for urothelial bladder cancer. Tumour Biol 2008;29:311–22.

27. Lee JT, Lehmann BD, Terrian DM, et al. Targeting prostate cancer based on signal transduction and cell cycle pathways. Cell Cycle 2008;7:1745–62.

28. Pruthi RS, Derksen JE, Moore D, et al. Phase II trial of celecoxib in prostate-specific antigen recurrent prostate cancer after definitive radiation therapy or radical prostatectomy. Clin Cancer Res 2006;12 (7 Pt 1):2172–7.

29. Smith MR, Manola J, Kaufman DS, et al. Celecoxib versus placebo for men with prostate cancer and a rising serum prostate-specific antigen after radical prostatectomy and/or radiation therapy. J Clin Oncol 2006;24:2723–8.

30. Kobayashi N, Barnard RJ, Henning SM, et al. Effect of altering dietary omega-6/omega-3 fatty acid ratios on prostate cancer membrane composition, cyclooxygenase-2, and prostaglandin E2. Clin Cancer Res 2006;12:4662–70.

31. Chan JM, Weinberg V, Magbanua MJ, et al. Nutritional supplements, COX-2 and IGF-1 expression in men on active surveillance for prostate cancer. Cancer Causes Control 2011;22:141–50.

32. Dimitrow PP, Jawien M. Pleiotropic, cardioprotective effects of omega-3 polyunsaturated fatty acids. Mini Rev Med Chem 2009;9:1030–9.

33. Reese AC, Fradet V, Witte JS. Omega-3 fatty acids, genetic variants in COX-2 and prostate cancer. J Nutrigenet Nutrigenomics 2009;2:149–58.

34. Lu X, Kang Y. Epidermal growth factor signaling and bone metastasis. Br J Cancer 2010;102:457–61.

35. Zhou T, Xu C, He M, et al. Upregulation of erythropoietin receptor in human prostate carcinoma and high-grade prostatic intraepithelial neoplasia. Prostate Cancer Prostatic Dis 2008;11:143–7.

36. Demark-Wahnefried W, Polascik TJ, George SL, et al. Flaxseed supplementation (not dietary fat restriction) reduces prostate cancer proliferation rates in men presurgery. Cancer Epidemiol Biomarkers Prev 2008;17:3577–87.

37. Lin Y, Wang F. FGF signaling in prostate development, tissue homoeostasis and tumorigenesis. Biosci Rep 2010;30:285–91.

38. Valta MP, Tuomela J, Bjartell A, et al. FGF-8 is involved in bone metastasis of prostate cancer. Int J Cancer 2008;123:22–31.

39. Gu F, Schumacher FR, Canzian F, et al. Eighteen insulin-like growth factor pathway genes, circulating levels of IGF-I and its binding protein, and risk of prostate and breast cancer. Cancer Epidemiol Biomarkers Prev 2010;19:2877–87.

40. Lima GA, Correa LL, Gabrich R, et al. IGF-I, insulin and prostate cancer. Arq Bras Endocrinol Metabol 2009;53:969–75.

41. Bouraoui Y, Ricote M, Garcia-Tunon I, et al. Pro-inflammatory cytokines and prostate-specific antigen in hyperplasia and human prostate cancer. Cancer Detect Prev 2008;32:23–32.

42. Waugh DJ, Wilson C. The interleukin-8 pathway in cancer. Clin Cancer Res 2008;14:6735–41.

43. Rao YK, Fang SH, Wu WS, et al. Constituents isolated from Cordyceps militaris suppress enhanced inflammatory mediator's production and human cancer cell proliferation. J Ethnopharmacol 2010;131:363–7.

44. Spencer L, Mann C, Metcalfe M, et al. The effect of omega-3 FAs on tumour angiogenesis and their therapeutic potential. Eur J Cancer 2009;45:2077–86.

45. Richardsen E, Uglehaus RD, Due J, et al. COX-2 is overexpressed in primary prostate cancer with metastatic potential and may predict survival. A comparison study between COX-2, TGF-beta, IL-10 and Ki67. Cancer Epidemiol 2010;34:316–22.

46. Grivennikov SI, Karin M. Inflammatory cytokines in cancer: tumour necrosis factor and interleukin 6 take the stage. Ann Rheum Dis 2011;70(Suppl 1):104–8.

47. Botelho F, Pina F, Lunet N. VEGF and prostatic cancer: a systematic review. Eur J Cancer Prev 2010;19:385–92.

48. Kosaka T, Miyajima A, Shirotake S, et al. Long-term androgen ablation and docetaxel up-regulate phosphorylated Akt in castration resistant prostate cancer. J Urol 2011;185(6):2376–81.

49. Neto AS, Tobias-Machado M, Wroclawski ML, et al. Molecular oncogenesis of prostate adenocarcinoma: role of the human epidermal growth factor receptor 2 (HER-2/neu). Tumori 2010;96:645–9.

50. Karin M. NF-kappaB as a critical link between inflammation and cancer. Cold Spring Harb Perspect Biol 2009;1:a000141.

Statin Clinical Trial (REALITY) for Prostate Cancer: an Over 15-Year Wait is Finally Over Thanks to a Dietary Supplement

Mark A. Moyad, MD, MPH[a,b,*], Laurence H. Klotz, MD[c]

KEYWORDS
- Prostate cancer • Red yeast rice • Statins • REALITY trial

Efforts to initiate a prospective study of cholesterol-lowering agents have been unsuccessful to date. Many designs, including the evaluation of lipid reduction for the prevention of prostate cancer in average and high-risk patients, for men with prostate cancer on active surveillance, or as a neoadjuvant or adjuvant treatment, have been proposed over the last 15 years. Lack of interest in such a trial has been due to multiple barriers, including: perceived lack of a compelling scientific rationale, concerns over unpredictable toxicity, lack of funding, corporate instability, competition from generics, and a perception that other micronutrients (vitamin E, selenium, and so forth) may be of more interest.[1–3]

However, over the last 7 years a great deal of epidemiologic and observational data has renewed interest in the relationship between cholesterol-lowering agents and prostate cancer progression.[4–17] The authors believe the time has come to formally evaluate this relationship in a prospective randomized trial.

RED YEAST RICE

The field of dietary supplements has evolved, and offers new opportunities for clinical trials. One such area is lipid-lowering treatment.[18] Most lipid-lowering dietary supplements are ineffective, particularly compared with pharmacologic statins.[18–21]

An important exception is red yeast rice (RYR) extract. This compound favorably competes with lovastatin, pravastatin, and simvastatin in terms of potency, and is a realistic alternative for statin-intolerant patients.[18,22–24] RYR has demonstrated a significant reduction in cardiovascular events (primary end point) in a randomized controlled trial of almost 5000 participants followed for a median of 4.5 years.[25]

RYR is a traditional Chinese herbal medicine first mentioned in 800 AD in the Tang Dynasty for blood circulation.[18,26,27] It is produced by the fermentation of the fungal strain *Monascus purpureus* Went (red yeast) over moist and sterile rice. RYR is also actually a common dietary compound and food colorant utilized in numerous Asian countries. In China, Japan, and several other countries it is used as an additive and preservative for fish and meat. It has a vibrant red color, flavor, and aroma, thus it is also used as a flavoring agent in several Chinese recipes and dishes, and is even used for brewing red rice wine. RYR is also known by several synonyms as

[a] Department of Urology, University of Michigan Medical Center, 1500 East Medical Center Drive , Ann Arbor, MI 48109-0330, USA
[b] Eisenhower Wellness Institute, Eisenhower Medical Center, Rancho Mirage, CA, USA
[c] Sunnybrook Health Science Centre, 2075 Bayview Avenue, #MG408, Toronto, ON M4N 3M5, Canada
* Corresponding author. Department of Urology, University of Michigan Medical Center, 1500 East Medical Center Drive, Ann Arbor, MI 48109-0330.
E-mail address: moyad@umich.edu

Urol Clin N Am 38 (2011) 325–331
doi:10.1016/j.ucl.2011.05.002
0094-0143/11/$ – see front matter © 2011 Elsevier Inc. All rights reserved.

a food product, including Hong Qu, Hung-Chu, Ang-kak, Ankak rice, red mold rice, and Beni-Koji.

In the late 1970s, Akira Endo[28] found that a Monascus yeast strain naturally produced a substance that inhibits cholesterol synthesis. He named it "monacolin K." This compound was later isolated and is now known to be of the same structure as lovastatin, the first marketed statin. Thus, RYR is the first statin used in medical history. Like RYR, a fungus, 3 of the first prescribed statins utilized in the United States were derived from fungi (lovastatin, pravastatin, and simvastatin).[18,29] Certain fungi use statin-like compounds to block the synthesis of cholesterol required by intruders (bacteria) for their cell wall synthesis, thus in part de-activating or eliminating the intruder. The analysis of this fascinating protective mechanism led to the isolation of a class of medications (statins) that have benefitted patients substantially. RYR contains 10 different compounds known as "monacolins" (statin-like compounds) that block the rate-limiting enzyme for cholesterol synthesis,[22,30] and these are listed in **Box 1**. Of these, Monacolin K is likely most responsible for the low-density lipoprotein (LDL) cholesterol reduction associated with RYR.

CLINICAL EFFICACY OF RYR

A meta-analysis of 9625 patients in 93 randomized trials involving 3 different commercial variants of RYR has summarized this large experience.[31] The mean reduction in total cholesterol, LDL cholesterol, triglyceride, and increase in high-density lipoprotein (HDL) cholesterol was respectively the following: −35 mg/dL (−0.91 mmol/L), −28 mg/dL (−0.73 mmol/L), −36 mg/dL (−0.41 mmol/L), and +6 mg/dL (+0.15 mmol/L).

Xuezhikang is a commercial RYR product evaluated in a large, randomized, placebo-controlled clinical trial with robust end points.[25,32] The China Coronary Secondary Prevention Study (CCSPS) enrolled 4870 participants (3986 men, 884 women) with a previous myocardial infarction (MI), and a baseline mean total cholesterol, LDL cholesterol, triglyceride, and HDL cholesterol of approximately 208 mg/dL (5.38 mmol/L), 129 mg/dL (3.34 mmol/L), 165 mg/dL (1.85 mmol/L), and 46 mg/dL (1.19 mmol/L). Participants received RYR, 600 mg twice daily (1200 mg total, monacolin K 2.5–3.2 mg/capsule) or matching placebo and were followed for 4.5 years. The trial was conducted from May 1996 to December 2003 in 65 hospitals in China. The primary end point was nonfatal MI or death from coronary or cardiac causes. Secondary end points included total mortality from cardiovascular disease, total all-cause mortality, need for coronary revascularization procedure, and change in lipid levels. Fasting blood samples were drawn at baseline, 6 to 8 weeks after randomization, and at 6-month intervals.

There were 2 interim analyses, and the second one demonstrated a significant difference for the primary end point. The study was stopped in June 2003. A total of 98% of the participants completed the study. Synopses of the results are found in **Tables 1** and **2**. It is of interest that a plethora of clinical end points were significantly reduced with the exception of a nonsignificant reduction in fatal MI. Cancer mortality and all-cause mortality were reduced. Lipids were also

Box 1
Monacolin compounds that can be detected in red yeast rice (RYR)
Dihydromonacolin K
Monacolin J
Monacolin JA
Monacolin K (lovastatin equivalent)
Monacolin KA
Monacolin L
Monacolin LA
Monacolin M
Monacolin X
Monacolin XA
Total monacolin content (sum of the 10 detectable monacolins)

Table 1		
Multiple clinical end-point observations in the largest randomized trial (CCSPS) of RYR		
Clinical End Points	**Risk Reduction (%) with RYR Compared with Placebo**	**P Value**
Nonfatal myocardial infarction	−62	<.001
Coronary disease death	−31	.005
Fatal myocardial infarction	−33	.19
Fatal stroke	−9	.85
Revascularization	−36	.004
Death from cardiovascular disease	−30	.005
Death from cancer	−56	.014
Total deaths	−33	.0003

Table 2
Lipid results in the largest randomized trial (CCSPS) of RYR

Lipid Value	Change (%) with RYR Compared with Placebo	P Value
Total cholesterol	−11	<.001
LDL cholesterol	−18	<.001
Triglycerides	−15	<.001
HDL cholesterol	+4.2	<.001

modestly and significantly reduced. No serious adverse events were observed during this trial. Total adverse events and treatment cessation numbers were similar for RYR and placebo. The number needed to treat (NNT) to prevent a primary end point over the 4.5-year duration of the trial is 21, which favorably compares with the NNT range (19–56) observed in previous secondary prevention trials.[33] Subsequent subgroup evaluations from the CCSPS trial have found equivalent benefits with RYR among diabetic,[34] elderly (mean age 69 years),[35] and hypertensive participants.[36] Potential anticancer benefits found in the overall trial with RYR were also found among the elderly (significant reduction in cancer deaths),[25,35] and included a 51% reduction in cancer incidence.[35] Thus, the data have been consistent in that RYR reduces lipid parameters, especially LDL,[37–39] and appears to have a favorable impact on clinical end points.[25]

A randomized trial of 74 dyslipidemia patients comparing 40 mg/d of simvastatin to a high-potency RYR (2.53 mg monacolin K per capsule, total monacolins, 5.3 mg/capsule) and lifestyle changes with fish oil found that the LDL reductions between both groups were similar after 12 weeks (−40% for simvastatin, −42% for RYR).[30] Participants consuming RYR needed to consume 4 to 6 capsules (2400–3600 mg RYR total) per day compared with 1 tablet per day for the prescription-drug group. No dropouts occurred, and there was no difference in adverse events reported. In the simvastatin arm 3 patients experienced musculoskeletal symptoms with 1 having elevated liver function tests (LFTs). RYR group had 1 patient with elevated creatine kinase numbers. This abnormality may have been caused by excessive exercise.

Another trial (N = 62) by the same principal author utilized a less potent RYR (1.02 mg monacolin K per capsule, total monacolins, 2.16 mg/capsule) at a dose of 6 capsules (3600 mg total RYR) per day compared with placebo for statin-intolerant (myalgia-induced) patients for 24 weeks and found a significant (P = .01) LDL reduction of −21.3%.[22] It should also be of interest that 93% of the subjects on RYR in this trial with a history of statin intolerance were able to tolerate this supplement without myalgia.

Another group of 43 statin-intolerant adults with dyslipidemia were randomized in a separate trial to prescription pravastatin at 20 mg (40 mg total) or RYR, 2400 mg twice daily (4800 mg total, monacolin K at 1.245 mg per capsule, 8 capsules/d), and both groups were asked to adhere to weekly healthy lifestyle educational sessions.[24] After 12 weeks a 30% reduction in LDL was observed for RYR and a 27% reduction for pravastatin. Only 1 of 21 in the RYR (5%) and 2 of 22 (9%) participants in the pravastatin group discontinued because of myalgia recurrence. Mean pain severity, and muscle strength at weeks 4, 8, and 12 did not differ. Other recent publications report similar results.[23,40] A recently published crossover study of children (aged 8–16 years) with heterozygous familial hypercholesterolemia (n = 24) and familial combined hyperlipidemia (n = 16) found that an RYR supplement significantly (P<.001) reduced LDL by 25%.[41] There were no adverse events in terms of liver or muscle enzyme abnormalities over the 8-week treatment period. The authors can propose multiple reasons for a low rate of toxicity with RYR overall in the literature (none proven): the diluted monacolin K in a supplement that contains mostly other ingredients, lower dose and potency of monacolin K/lovastatin compared with the previous statin utilized, multiple capsules during the day compared with one bolus at one specific time, which reduces the risk of excessive blood concentrations or impact with CYP3A4 inhibitors, other compounds that may deter myalgia in RYR (coenzyme Q–like effects), lack of aggressive monitoring, the desire to report fewer side effects from patients on a supplement compared with a drug, and so forth.

Prostate Cancer

RYR has direct effects on androgen-dependent LNCaP cells and androgen-independent cells over expressing androgen receptor.[42] RYR inhibited prostate cancer growth compared with a prescription statin (lovastatin). Whole RYR inhibited proliferation to a greater extent than monacolin K and pigment-enriched fractions isolated from RYR (P<.001). These results suggested that intact RYR, beyond the monacolin content, may favorably inhibit androgen-dependent and androgen-independent prostate cancer growth. A recent study showed that RYR significantly reduced androgen-dependent and androgen-independent xenograft tumors in SCID mice ($P<.05$).[43] Intact whole RYR again provided more inhibition than monacolin K alone. RYR also significantly ($P<.05$) reduced gene expression of several androgen-synthesizing enzymes (AKR1C3, HSD3B2, and SRD5A1) in both androgen-dependent and androgen-independent tumors. A significant ($P<.001$) association was seen between tumor volume and serum cholesterol. Similar findings have been demonstrated in colon cancer cell lines.[44] Other studies have demonstrated that RYR has pleiotropic actions on a variety of pathways and markers beyond LDL cholesterol,[45–48] which could have an impact on prostate cancer proliferation and progression.[49–51] Thus RYR has the appeal of an inexpensive nontoxic natural compound that is equivalent to many statins and may have further inhibitory effects on prostate cancer.

The authors believe that the active surveillance population is ideal for an initial clinical trial of RYR.[7,52] Repeat biopsy and prostate-specific antigen kinetic data can be gleaned rapidly without the interference of other treatment manipulations. In addition, a preventive agent that is heart healthy and can prevent the progression of a minimal-volume low-grade tumor to a more clinically significant disease would be of enormous value in this population of men. Heart disease is the number one cause of mortality in men with prostate cancer, so an agent that simultaneously improved heart and prostate health in active surveillance patients is a rational choice.[7] The observational data suggest that if statins provide benefit, they do so by preventing progression or transformation to an aggressive disease state. One literature review stated

> One interesting option that could be used to study the efficacy of statins in the prevention of prostate cancer is a randomized clinical trial that includes men with localized and well-differentiated prostate cancer who have chosen to be managed by active surveillance instead of intervention. Such patients could be randomly allocated to receive either a statin or placebo, with disease progression as the study end point. This kind of trial is made possible by the currently increasing trend for active surveillance to be considered as an acceptable management strategy for small, well-differentiated, prostate tumors.[52]

The quotation referred to ongoing data on active surveillance from Klotz.[53]

The authors will be conducting their trial in Toronto, Canada. Men will receive 3600 mg daily of RYR with a potency of monacolin K that is approximately 2.5 mg per capsule, based on previous clinical trials. It is expected that compliant participants will experience a 20% to 35% LDL-cholesterol reduction. Active surveillance patients will be followed for at least 1 year and have at least 2 biopsies in this 12-month period.[54,55] The level of LDL is not predictive for response, and therefore will not be an eligibility criterion.

LIMITATIONS OF RYR

Quality control with this over-the-counter product is an issue.[56–59] Different commercial products of RYR have different concentrations of monacolins. Some contain a potentially harmful by-product of yeast fermentation known as "citrinin."[59] The REALITY trial will contain a monacolin K content similar to that used in the largest randomized trial of RYR, and be confirmed to be void of citrinin and other contaminants.

RYR has been promoted as a safe and effective alternative to statins.[60–63] Myopathy on statins is not a contraindication to RYR.[22–24,60–63] However, RYR requires medical oversight. Case reports of hepatotoxicity,[64,65] myopathy,[66–71] and rhabdomyolysis have been reported.[72] The contraindications for RYR should be similar to lovastatin, including hepatic or renal impairment, and allergies to yeast or fungus. RYR should be taken with or especially after meals, because lovastatin absorption is significantly improved under these circumstances, but only as long as pectin or oat bran (high fiber) is not consumed with it because these products specifically reduce absorption.[73–75] There has been no consistent mention of this potentially positive and negative interaction with RYR and food in the medical literature or data relating to RYR specifically (only lovastatin).

SUMMARY

RYR is a safe, inexpensive, widely used natural compound, which acts as an effective statin and appears to inhibit prostate cancer proliferation in preclinical studies. It is very compelling as a preventive agent for both heart disease and prostate cancer. The active surveillance population is ideally suited for evaluating the effect of this agent on prostate cancer progression.

REFERENCES

1. van Adelsberg J, Gann P, Ko AT, et al. The VIOXX in Prostate Cancer Prevention study: cardiovascular events observed in the rofecoxib 25 mg and placebo treatment groups. Curr Med Res Opin 2007;23:2063–70.

2. Thompson IM, Tangen CM, Klein EA, et al. Phase III prostate cancer prevention trials: are the costs justified? J Clin Oncol 2005;23:8161–4.

3. Klein EA, Thompson IM, Lippman SM, et al. SELECT: the next prostate cancer prevention trial. Selenium and Vitamin E Cancer Prevention Trial. J Urol 2001; 166:1311–5.

4. Moyad MA. Heart healthy equals prostate healthy equals statins: the next cancer chemoprevention trial. Part I. Curr Opin Urol 2005;15:1–6.

5. Moyad MA. Why a statin and/or another proven heart healthy agent should be utilized in the next major cancer chemoprevention trial: part I. Urol Oncol 2004;22:466–71.

6. Moyad MA. Why a statin and/or another proven heart healthy agent should be utilized in the next major cancer chemoprevention trial: part II. Urol Oncol 2004;22:472–7.

7. Moyad MA, Merrick GS. Statins and cholesterol lowering after a cancer diagnosis: why not? Urol Oncol 2005;23:49–55.

8. Moyad MA, Merrick GS, Butler WM, et al. Statins, especially atorvastatin, may favorably influence clinical presentation and biochemical progression-free survival after brachytherapy for clinically localized prostate cancer. Urology 2005;66:1150–4.

9. Shannon J, Tewoderos S, Garzotto M, et al. Statins and prostate cancer risk: a case-control study. Am J Epidemiol 2005;162:318–25.

10. Cyrus-David MS, Weinberg A, Thompson T, et al. The effect of statins on serum prostate specific antigen levels in a cohort of airline pilots: a preliminary report. J Urol 2005;173:1923–5.

11. Zhuang L, Kim J, Adam RM, et al. Cholesterol targeting alters lipid raft composition and cell survival in prostate cancer cells and xenografts. J Clin Invest 2005;115:959–68.

12. Platz EA, Leitzmann MF, Visvanathan K, et al. Statin drugs and risk of advanced prostate cancer. J Natl Cancer Inst 2006;98:1819–25.

13. Jacobs EJ, Rodriguez C, Bain EB, et al. Cholesterol-lowering drugs and advanced prostate cancer incidence in a large U.S. cohort. Cancer Epidemiol Biomarkers Prev 2007;16:2213–7.

14. Colli JL, Amling CL. Exploring causes for declining prostate cancer mortality rates in the United States. Urol Oncol 2008;26:627–33.

15. Murtola TJ, Pennanen P, Syvala H, et al. Effects of simvastatin, acetylsalicylic acid, and rosiglitazone on proliferation of normal and cancerous prostate epithelial cells at therapeutic concentrations. Prostate 2009;69:1017–23.

16. Loeb S, Kan D, Helfand BT, et al. Is statin use associated with prostate cancer aggressiveness? BJU Int 2010;105:1222–5.

17. Farwell WR, D'Avolio LW, Scranton RE, et al. Statins and prostate cancer diagnosis and grade in a Veterans population. J Natl Cancer Inst 2011; 103:885–92.

18. Nijjar PS, Burke FM, Bloesch A, et al. Role of dietary supplements in lowering low-density lipoprotein cholesterol: a review. J Clin Lipidol 2010;4:248–58.

19. Marinangeli CP, Jones PJ, Kassis AN, et al. Policosanols as nutraceuticals: fact or fiction. Crit Rev Food Sci Nutr 2010;50:259–67.

20. Khoo YS, Aziz Z. Garlic supplementation and serum cholesterol: a meta-analysis. J Clin Pharm Ther 2009;34:133–45.

21. Thompson Coon JS, Ernst E. Herbs for serum cholesterol reduction: a systematic review. J Fam Pract 2003;52:468–78.

22. Becker DJ, Gordon RY, Halbert SC, et al. Red yeast rice for dyslipidemia in statin-intolerant patients: a randomized trial. Ann Intern Med 2009;150:830–9.

23. Venero CV, Venero JV, Wortham DC, et al. Lipid-lowering efficacy of red yeast rice in a population intolerant to statins. Am J Cardiol 2010;105:664–6.

24. Halbert SC, French B, Gordon RY, et al. Tolerability of red yeast rice (2400 mg twice daily) versus pravastatin (20 mg twice daily) in patients with previous statin intolerance. Am J Cardiol 2010;105:198–204.

25. Lu Z, Kou W, Du B, et al, Chinese Coronary Secondary Prevention Group. Effects of Xuezhikang, an extract from red yeast Chinese rice, on coronary events in a Chinese population with previous myocardial infarction. Am J Cardiol 2008;101:1689–93.

26. Li C, Zhu Y, Wang Y, et al. Monascus purpureus fermented rice (red yeast rice): a natural food product that lowers blood cholesterol in animal models of hypercholesterolemia. Nutr Res 1998;18:71–81. Red yeast rice. Med Lett Drugs Ther 2009;51:71–2.

27. Lin Y-L, Wang T-H, Lee M-H, et al. Biologically active components and nutraceuticals in the Monascus-fermented rice: a review. Appl Microbiol Biotechnol 2008;77:965–73.

28. Endo A. Monacolin K, a new hypocholesterolemic agent produced by a Monascus species. J Antibiot (Tokyo) 1979;32:852–4.

29. Landers P. Stalking cholesterol. How one scientist intrigued by molds found first statin. Feat of Japan's Dr. Endo led to heart-care revolution but brought him nothing. Nature as a drug laboratory. Wall Street Journal. New York: Dow Jones and Company; 2006. p. A1, A8.

30. Becker DJ, Gordon RY, Morris PB, et al. Simvastatin vs therapeutic lifestyle changes and supplements: randomized primary prevention trial. Mayo Clin Proc 2008;83:758–64.

31. Liu J, Zhang J, Shi Y, et al. Chinese red yeast rice (Monascus purpureus) for primary hyperlipidemia: a meta-analysis of randomized controlled trials. Chin Med 2006;1:4.

32. China Coronary Secondary Prevention Study Group. China coronary secondary prevention study

(CCSPS)-lipid regulating therapy with xuezhikang for secondary prevention of coronary heart disease. Chin J Cardiol (Chin) 2005;33:109–15.

33. Ong HT. The statin studies: from targeting hypercholesterolemia to targeting the high risk patient. QJM 2005;98:599–614.

34. Zhao SP, Lu ZL, Du BM, et al, China Coronary Secondary Prevention Study. Xuezhikang, an extract of cholestin, reduces cardiovascular events in type 2 diabetes patients with coronary heart disease: subgroup analysis of patients with type 2 diabetes from Chian coronary secondary prevention study (CCSPS). J Cardiovasc Pharmacol 2007;49:81–4.

35. Ye P, Lu ZL, Du BM, et al, CCSPS Investigators. Effects of xuezhikang on cardiovascular events and mortality in elderly patients with a history of myocardial infarction: a subgroup analysis of elderly subjects from China coronary secondary prevention study. J Am Geriatr Soc 2007;55:1015–22.

36. Li JJ, Lu ZL, Kou WR, et al, Chinese Coronary Secondary Prevention Study (CCSPS) Group. Long-term effects of Xuezhikang on blood pressure in hypertensive patients with previous myocardial infarction: data from the Chinese Coronary Secondary Prevention Study (CCSPS). Clin Exp Hypertens 2010;32(8):491–8.

37. Huang CF, Li TC, Lin CC, et al. Efficacy of *Monascus purpureus* Went rice on lowering lipid ratios in hypercholesterolemic patients. Eur J Cardiovasc Prev Rehabil 2007;14:438–40.

38. Lin CC, Li TC, Lai MM. Efficacy and safety of *Monascus purpureus* Went rice in subjects with hyperlipidemia. Eur J Endocrinol 2005;153:679–86.

39. Heber D, Yip I, Ashley JM, et al. Cholesterol-lowering effects of a proprietary Chinese red-yeast-rice dietary supplement. Am J Clin Nutr 1999;69:231–6.

40. Bogsrud MP, Ose L, Langslet G, et al. HypoCol (red yeast rice) lowers plasma cholesterol-a randomized placebo controlled study. Scand Cardiovasc J 2010; 44:197–200.

41. Guardamagna O, Abello F, Baracco V, et al. The treatment of hypercholesterolemic children: Efficacy and safety of a combination of red yeast rice extract and policosanols. Nutr Metab Cardiovasc Dis 2011; 21:424–9.

42. Hong MY, Seeram NP, Zhang Y, et al. Chinese red yeast rice versus lovastatin effects on prostate cancer cells with and without androgen receptor overexpression. J Med Food 2008;11:657–66.

43. Hong MY, Henning S, Moro A, et al. Chinese red yeast rice inhibition of prostate tumor growth in SCID mice. Cancer Prev Res (Phila) 2011;4:608–15.

44. Hong MY, Seeram NP, Zhang Y, et al. Anticancer effects of Chinese red yeast rice versus monacolin K alone on colon cancer cells. J Nutr Biochem 2008;19:448–58.

45. Ma KY, Zhang ZS, Zhao SX, et al. Red yeast increases excretion of bile acids in hamsters. Biomed Environ Sci 2009;22:269–77.

46. Li JJ, Hu SS, Fang CH, et al. Effects of xuezhikang, an extract of cholestin, on lipid profile and C-reactive protein: a short-term time course study in patients with stable angina. Clin Chim Acta 2005; 352:217–24.

47. Zhao SP, Liu L, Cheng YC, et al. Xuezhikang, an extract of cholestin, protects endothelial function through anti-inflammatory and lipid-lowering mechanisms in patients with coronary heart disease. Circulation 2004;110:915–20.

48. Liu L, Zhao SP, Cheng YC, et al. Xuezhikang decreases serum lipoprotein(a) and C-reactive protein concentrations in patients with coronary heart disease. Clin Chem 2003;49:1347–52.

49. Eisberger B, Lankston L, McMillan DC, et al. Presence of tumoural C-reactive protein correlates with progressive prostate cancer. Prostate Cancer Prostatic Dis 2011;14:122–8.

50. Lehrer S, Diamond EJ, Mamkine B, et al. C-reactive protein is significantly associated with prostate-specific antigen and metastatic disease in prostate cancer. BJU Int 2005;95:961–2.

51. Solomon KR, Pelton K, Boucher K, et al. Ezetimibe is an inhibitor if tumor angiogenesis. Am J Pathol 2009; 174:1017–26.

52. Murtola TJ, Visakorpi T, Lahtela J, et al. Statins and prostate cancer prevention: where we are now, and future directions. Nat Clin Pract Urol 2008;5:376–87.

53. Klotz L. Active surveillance versus radical treatment for favorable-risk localized prostate cancer. Curr Treat Options Oncol 2006;7:355–62.

54. Gotto AM Jr, Whitney E, Stein EA, et al. Relation between baseline and on treatment lipid parameters and first major acute major coronary events in the Air Force/Texas Coronary Atherosclerosis Prevention Study (AFCAPS/TexCAPS). Circulation 2000;101: 477–84.

55. Nakamura H; MEGA Study Group. Primary prevention of cardiovascular diseases among hypercholesterolemic Japanese with a low dose of pravastatin. Atheroscler Suppl 2007;8:13–7.

56. Gordon RY, Cooperman T, Obermeyer W, et al. Marked variability of monacolin levels in commercial red yeast rice products: buyer beware. Arch Intern Med 2010;170:1722–7.

57. Harding A. Contamination common in red yeast rice products. New York: Thompson Reuters; 2008. Available at: www.reuters.com/article/healthNews/idUSCOL97022820080709. Accessed April 25, 2011.

58. Klimek M, Wang S, Ogunkanmi A. Safety and efficacy of red yeast rice (*Monascus purpureus*) as an alternative therapy for hyperlipidemia. P T 2009; 34:313–27.

59. Heber D, Lembertas A, Lu QY, et al. An analysis of nine proprietary Chinese red yeast rice dietary supplements: implications of variability in chemical profile and contents. J Altern Complement Med 2001;7:133–9.

60. Abd TT, Jacobson TA. Statin-induced myopathy: a review and update. Expert Opin Drug Saf 2011; 10:373–87.

61. Eckel RH. Approach to the patient who is intolerant of statin therapy. J Clin Endocrinol Metab 2010;95: 2015–22.

62. Kelly RB. Diet and exercise in the management of hyperlipidemia. Am Fam Physician 2010;81: 1097–102.

63. Lin JS. An alternative treatment of hyperlipidemia with red yeast rice: a case report. J Med Case Reports 2010;4:4.

64. Roselle H, Ekatan A, Tzeng J, et al. Symptomatic hepatitis associated with the use of herbal red yeast rice [letter]. Ann Intern Med 2008;149:516–7.

65. Grieco A, Miele L, Pompili M, et al. Acute hepatitis caused by a natural lipid-lowering product: when "alternative" medicine is no "alternative" at all. J Hepatol 2009;50:1273–7.

66. Polsani VR, Jones PH, Ballantyne CM, et al. A case report of myopathy from consumption of red yeast rice. J Clin Lipidol 2008;2:60–2.

67. Lapi F, Gallo E, Bernasconi S, et al. Myopathies associated with red yeast rice and liquorice: spontaneous reports from the Italian Surveillance System of Natural Health Products [letter]. Br J Clin Pharmacol 2008;66:572–4.

68. Mueller PS. Symptomatic myopathy due to red yeast rice [letter]. Ann Intern Med 2006;145:474–5.

69. Smith DJ, Olive KE. Chinese red rice-induced myopathy. South Med J 2003;96:1265–7.

70. Vercelli L, Mongini T, Olivero N, et al. Chinese red rice depletes muscle coenzyme Q10 and maintains muscle damage after discontinuation of statin treatment [letter]. J Am Geriatr Soc 2006;54:718–20.

71. Cartin-Ceba R, Lu LB, Kolpakchi A. A "natural" threat [letter]. Am J Med 2007;120:e3–4.

72. Prasad GV, Wong T, Meliton G, et al. Rhabdomyolysis due to red yeast rice (Monascus purpureus) in a renal transplant recipient. Transplantation 2002;74:1200–1.

73. Garnett WR. Interactions with hydroxymethylglutaryl-coenzyme A reductase inhibitors. Am J Health Syst Pharm 1995;52:1639–45.

74. Schacter M. Chemical, pharmacokinetic and pharmacodynamic properties of statins: an update. Fundam Clin Pharmacol 2005;19:117–25.

75. Moghadasian MH. Clinical pharmacology of 3-hydroxy-3-methylglutaryl coenzyme A reductase inhibitors. Life Sci 1999;65:1329–37.

Prostate Cancer and Vitamin D: What Does the Evidence Really Suggest?

Christine M. Barnett, MD*, Tomasz M. Beer, MD

KEYWORDS

• Prostate cancer • Vitamin D • Supplementation • UV

At present, the optimal approach to vitamin D supplementation for the average healthy person is debated. In patients with cancer, the role of vitamin D supplementation in treatment, is even less clear. With the recent publication of new guidelines by the Institute of Medicine (IOM) for vitamin D supplementation, the question how much vitamin D a human requires arises. For years, many physicians have been recommending vitamin D supplementation at doses somewhat higher than national recommendations because evidence had suggested that vitamin D may play a role in the prevention and treatment of several diseases. The hypothesis that this evidence suggests has been of significant interest to cancer researchers.

For decades, there have been efforts to test the hypothesis that low vitamin D plays a role in prostate cancer development and progression.[1] Epidemiologic observations show that populations in areas with low UV exposure have an increased risk of prostate cancer,[2–7] and laboratory experiments showing antitumor effects of vitamin D have provided evidence supporting this hypothesis and have stimulated further studies examining the relationship between prostate cancer and vitamin D in humans. However, studies looking for a direct association between serum vitamin D levels and prostate cancer have not consistently supported this hypothesis. In addition, the use of vitamin D as a therapeutic addition to prostate cancer treatments has not achieved consistently positive results to date.

VITAMIN D BIOLOGY

Vitamin D acts as a regulatory hormone for multiple cell activities in the human body. The activated form of vitamin D is 1,25-OH$_2$ vitamin D, which is formed through several tightly regulated synthesis steps (**Fig. 1**). The process begins with 7-deoxycholesterol that is converted to pre–vitamin D in the presence of UV-B light. The 7-deoxycholesterol is then converted to 25-OH vitamin D, the main circulating form of vitamin D in the body, by the enzyme 25-hydroxylase, predominantly in the liver. The final conversion to 1,25-OH$_2$ vitamin D, which is catalyzed by 1α-hydroxylase, primarily occurs in the kidney but can also be seen in other tissues such as the prostate,[8,9] which can potentially play a role in cancer pathogenesis.

The vitamin D receptor (VDR) is a steroid receptor. When bound by 1,25-OH$_2$ vitamin D, the VDR is translocated to the nucleus to regulate gene expression (**Fig. 2**). In this way, the VDR acts as a ligand-activated (1,25-OH$_2$ vitamin D) transcription factor. Once activated, the VDR forms a heterodimer with retinoid-X receptor, which aids in binding the receptor complex to DNA. The activated VDR then binds to the promoter region of specific genes with vitamin D response elements (VDREs) and regulates the transcription

Division of Hematology and Medical Oncology, Knight Cancer Institute, Oregon Health and Science University, Mail Code L586, 3181 Southwest Sam Jackson Park Road, Portland, OR 97239, USA
* Corresponding author.
E-mail address: barnetch@ohsu.edu

Urol Clin N Am 38 (2011) 333–342
doi:10.1016/j.ucl.2011.04.007
0094-0143/11/$ – see front matter © 2011 Elsevier Inc. All rights reserved.

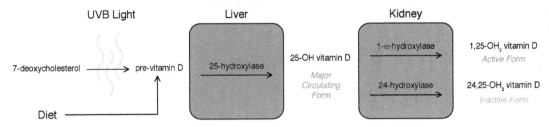

Fig. 1. Vitamin D synthesis.

of messenger RNA in these genes. The regulatory effect of vitamin D on calcium through transcriptional regulation of genes such as osteocalcin[10] and PTH is well established, but additional genes with VDREs are increasingly being discovered. For example, cell cycle regulators, such as p21,[11] Bcl-2,[12] and insulinlike growth factor,[13] and cell signaling molecules, such as tumor necrosis factor α[14] and epidermal growth factor receptor,[15] have been found to have VDREs. The transcriptional regulation, either upregulation or downregulation, of these genes is the basis for the observed experimental antineoplastic effects of vitamin D. Nongenomic direct actions of the VDR on cell signaling and growth have also been described.

VITAMIN D ANTI–PROSTATE CANCER ACTIVITY

With many cell cycle regulatory genes having VDREs, multiple studies have focused on examining the potential antitumor activity of vitamin D in different tumor models. There have been multiple examples of vitamin D–induced cell cycle arrest in G1 and inhibition of mitosis induction pathways.[11,16] There have also been VDRs demonstrated on prostate carcinoma cell lines.[17,18] In cell

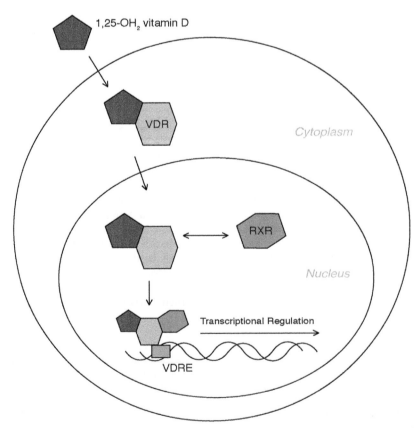

Fig. 2. Vitamin D–regulated gene transcription. VDRE, vitamin D response element; RXR, retinoid-X receptor.

lines,[18] cell culture,[19] and mouse models,[20] vitamin D has been shown to have antiproliferative and, therefore, antineoplastic actions.

A question that arises is why have these antineoplastic effects of vitamin D not been consistently seen with prostate cancer in human experience, although they have been shown in the laboratory. One hypothesis is based on the ability of prostate cells to locally activate $1,25$-OH_2 vitamin D from 25-OH vitamin D through the enzymatic activity of 1α-hydroxylase.

Normal prostate cells have been found to express 1α-hydroxylase.[8,9] As mentioned, most activations to $1,25$-OH_2 vitamin D occur in the kidney, so why would prostate cells need to express their own 1α-hydroxylase? Perhaps the ability of the prostate cell to locally activate vitamin D is important for normal cell regulation. It has been shown that prostate cancer cells lose the activity of 1α-hydroxlase in the laboratory.[8,21] However, this phenomenon has not been fully characterized in humans. Loss of local 1α-hydroxylase may render prostate cancer cells more dependent on circulating $1,25$-OH_2 vitamin D rather than on the more abundant precursor 25-OH vitamin D, which can reduce the prostate cell's ability to regulate its own growth in response to vitamin D levels. To demonstrate this finding, restoring 1α-hydroxylase activity in LNCaP cells with gene transfer has been shown to restore the antineoplastic effects of 25-OH vitamin D.[22]

Because $1,25$-OH_2 vitamin D levels are usually tightly regulated and only decrease during severe deficiency states, tissues that rely on renally activated vitamin D are relatively unaffected by mild vitamin D deficiency states. However, tissues, such as the prostate, that may rely on local production of $1,25$-OH_2 vitamin D could experience decreased VDR signaling with small changes in 25-OH vitamin D levels, which are more closely linked to a patient's overall vitamin D status. The decreased 1α-hydroxlase activity in prostate cancer cells should render the cells more free to proliferate in states without adequate circulating 25-OH vitamin D levels. This finding is yet to be demonstrated in human studies measuring 25-OH vitamin D serum levels, and it is therefore not known if the changes in local vitamin D synthetic capacity observed in models of prostate carcinogenesis are important in the human disease.

PROSTATE CANCER AND VITAMIN D: EPIDEMIOLOGIC EVIDENCE

There are multiple laboratory studies showing that vitamin D can play a role in prostate cancer biology, but what evidence is there in humans to confirm that vitamin D can have an appreciable effect on prostate cancer development or progression?

UV Exposure Data

The hypothesis that vitamin D may play a role in cancer biology was formed after geographic studies demonstrated that there may be an increased risk of dying from cancer in areas with low UV exposure.[2] This geographic distribution of cancer-related mortality, with the highest risk in northern regions, was seen in a variety of cancers, including prostate cancer (**Table 1**). The initial studies, from the early 1990s, have been confirmed in later geographic studies as well.[3–7] In addition to an increased prostate cancer mortality based on geographic location, cancer mortality risk has also been shown to have seasonal variations. Two recent studies have shown that there is a decreased risk of prostate cancer death when a patient is diagnosed in the summer, both showing a relative risk reduction of approximately 20%.[23,24]

Of the 8 studies performed that examined markers of UV exposure, an impressive 75% returned a result linking reduced UV exposure to increased prostate cancer risk or increased prostate cancer–related mortality. Further, the 2 studies that did not show a geographically linked increased prostate cancer risk[23,24] did show a difference in mortality for season of diagnosis.

Dietary and Supplement Data

There are multiple feedback loops that regulate the activation of $1,25$-OH_2 vitamin D. One of these feedback loops includes high serum calcium levels acting to reduce the activity of 1α-hydroxylase, which in turn reduces the synthesis of active $1,25$-OH_2 vitamin D, thus decreasing the absorption of calcium. With this in mind, it would be expected that high calcium intake could have a detrimental effect on active vitamin D production and, thus, an increased risk of prostate cancer if the UV exposure hypothesis is correct. However, this finding has not been shown consistently across multiple studies. There have been 12 recent studies comparing calcium and vitamin D intake and the risk of developing prostate cancer (**Table 2**). Of these studies, 8 showed no association with calcium intake (variously defined) and prostate cancer risk.[25–32] Of those eight studies, 2 showed an association with one form of calcium intake and prostate cancer risk but not another. One found an association with total calcium and dietary intake but not with supplemental calcium intake.[25] One study even showed a decreased risk of prostate cancer with higher calcium intake.[33] There were, however, 6 studies that

Table 1
Studies of UV exposure and prostate cancer

Study	Year	Location	Measure	If Low UV Exposure is Associated with Increased Prostate Cancer Risk or Mortality
Hanchette[2]	1992	United States	Scored locations in the United States based on a combination of cloud cover, latitude, and altitude	Yes, increased mortality
Luscombe[3]	2001	United Kingdom	Sunbathing score	Yes, increased risk
Grant[4]	2002	United States	Scored locations in the United States based on UV-B radiation map	Yes, increased mortality
Bodiwala[5]	2003	United Kingdom	Sunbathing score	Yes, increased risk
John[6]	2005	Western United States	Measured skin pigmentation	Yes, increased risk (of advanced prostate cancer)
Schwartz[7]	2006	United States	UV index data	Yes, increased mortality
Robsahm[23]	2004	Norway	Scored regions in Norway based on latitude and climate	No[a]
Lagunova[24]	2007	Norway	Annual ambient UV exposure and incidence of squamous cell carcinoma of the skin	No[b]

[a] Diagnosis of prostate cancer in autumn was associated with decreased mortality (relative risk, 0.83).
[b] Diagnosis of prostate cancer in summer and autumn was associated with decreased mortality (relative risk, 0.8).

showed some increased prostate cancer risk with increased calcium intake.[25,26,34–37] These results could be explained by differences in calcium absorption. A study that had measured serum calcium levels to clarify this result[37] showed an increased risk of death caused by prostate cancer with higher serum calcium levels. Serum calcium level, however, is not a strong indicator of calcium intake because it reflects the homeostatic balance of calcium exchange within the bone matrix, renal calcium handling, as well as intake and absorption. None of these 12 studies showed a link between vitamin D intake and prostate cancer risk.

Serum Data

A possible reason for the more-consistent association seen in the UV studies and not in the dietary studies is that UV exposure affects vitamin D levels more profoundly than calcium intake or vitamin D supplementation does. If this were the case, an association between vitamin D and prostate cancer should be able to be demonstrated by studies directly measuring serum vitamin D in patients. Serum-based studies are the best at measuring overall vitamin D status. Because of

the tight control of renal 1α-hydroxylase, there is less variability in $1,25\text{-OH}_2$ vitamin D levels. Further, it is not clear to what extent serum assessment reflects tissue vitamin D status, particularly in tumor tissues. Many of the studies examined vitamin D levels at a single point in time or limited number of time points and, therefore, may not adequately capture long-term vitamin D status of patients. Long-term status may be important in patients with malignancies, such as prostate cancer, that have a prolonged gestational period, that is, decades.

There have been 13 case-cohort or case-control studies measuring serum vitamin D levels and correlating these levels with the risk of prostate cancer (**Table 3**). About 70% of these studies did not find the expected association between low vitamin D levels and increased risk of prostate cancer. One of the studies with positive results, which demonstrated an increased risk of prostate cancer with low 25-OH levels, also showed an increased risk with high 25-OH levels.[38] Another study that did not show an association with low 25-OH levels did show an increased risk of aggressive prostate cancer with high 25-OH levels.[39] This finding has not been consistently demonstrated in

Table 2
Studies of dietary calcium and vitamin D and prostate cancer risk

Study	Year	Number of Subjects	Age (y)	Diet/Supplementation	Is There Association with Prostate Cancer Risk
Chan[35]	1998	1062	<80	Calcium and dairy intake	Yes, increased risk
Giovannucci[48]	1998	1792	40–75	Dietary and supplementary calcium	Yes, increased risk of aggressive and metastatic prostate cancer
Skinner[37]	2008	2814	24–77	Serum calcium	Yes, increased risk
Kristal[33]	2010	9559	>55	Calcium intake	Yes, decreased risk of high-grade prostate cancer
				Vitamin D intake	No
Ahn[25]	2007	29,509	55–74	Dietary calcium	Yes, increased risk
				Supplemental calcium	No
Rodriguez[26]	2003	65,321	50–74	Total calcium intake	Yes, increased risk
				Dairy intake	No
Kristal[34]	2002	605	40–64	Calcium intake	Yes, increased risk of aggressive prostate cancer
				Vitamin D intake	No
Park[27]	2007	10,180	50–71	Calcium intake	No
Chan[28]	2000	27,111	50–69	Calcium intake	No
Baron[29,a]	2005	672	61.8 (mean)	Calcium supplementation	No
Berndt[30]	2002	454	46–92	Calcium intake	No
Tavani[32]	2005	2745	46–74	Calcium intake	No
				Vitamin D intake	No
Tavani[31]	2001	1050	45–79	Calcium intake	No

[a] Only randomized controlled trial.

other studies and needs further investigation but brings up the question of whether or not more vitamin D is always better.

Of the 4 studies with positive results, only 2 found an association between increased prostate cancer risk and low levels of 25-OH vitamin D if $1,25\text{-OH}_2$ vitamin D levels were also low. This result suggests that low 25-OH vitamin D levels may not increase prostate cancer risk or aggressiveness unless it is low enough to affect circulating $1,25\text{-OH}_2$ vitamin D levels. The aforementioned prostate cell dependence on its own 1α-hydroxylase to produce local $1,25\text{-OH}_2$ vitamin D along with the loss of this enzyme in prostate cancer seems to make the prostate cell sensitive to only small changes in 25-OH vitamin D levels. However, extrarenal 1α-hydroxylase has been shown to be constitutively active and not downregulated by $1,25\text{-OH}_2$ vitamin D. Therefore, if the lack of activated $1,25\text{-OH}_2$ vitamin D causes cancer proliferation in the prostate, little effect is expected from low 25-OH vitamin D levels unless circulating $1,25\text{-OH}_2$ vitamin D levels were also affected.

This may explain why most studies in which more than 50% of the patients had vitamin D deficiency showed an increased risk of prostate cancer with low vitamin D levels. This finding may indicate that unless 25-OH vitamin D is very low, there will not be an effect on prostate cancer risk. However, most studies measuring both 25-OH vitamin D and $1,25\text{-OH}_2$ vitamin D levels did not show an association between low levels and an increased risk of prostate cancer.

There is a possibility that these case-control and case-cohort studies did not examine enough patients with severe vitamin D deficiency to detect an effect or that prostate tissue levels of vitamin D are more clinically important than serum vitamin D status. In addition, it seems that if a link does exist, there may be an increased risk of more aggressive prostate cancers rather than an increase in prostate cancer incidence in low vitamin D states.

Table 3
Case-cohort and case-control studies measuring serum vitamin D and prostate cancer risk

Study	Year	Population/Location	Age (y)	Number of Patients	Vitamin D Deficiency[a] (%)	Measure	Is Low Vitamin D Associated with Increased Prostate Cancer Risk or Mortality
Corder[49]	1993	United States	38–89	181	Approximately 50	$1,25\text{-}OH_2$ / $25\text{-}OH$	Yes, increased risk with low $1,25\text{-}OH_2$ levels, especially with concurrent low $25\text{-}OH$ levels
Ahonen[50]	2000	Finland	40–55	149	>60	$25\text{-}OH$	Yes, increased risk of aggressive cancer
Tuohimaa[38]	2004	Scandinavia	40–58	622	Approximately 50	$25\text{-}OH$	Yes, increased risk[c]
Li[51]	2007	United States	40–84	492	19	$1,25\text{-}OH_2$ / $25\text{-}OH$	Yes, increased risk of aggressive cancer with low $1,25\text{-}OH_2$ levels, especially with concurrent low $25\text{-}OH$ levels
Braun[52]	1995	White	—	61	Approximately 10	$1,25\text{-}OH_2$ / $25\text{-}OH$	No
Gann[53]	1996	United States	40–84	232	Approximately 20	$1,25\text{-}OH_2$	No[b]
Nomura[54]	1998	US Asians	45–68	136	None	$1,25\text{-}OH_2$ / $25\text{-}OH$	No
Platz[55]	2004	United States	40–75	460	Approximately 20	$1,25\text{-}OH_2$ / $25\text{-}OH$	No
Jacobs[56]	2004	Eastern United States	67.2 (mean)	83	20	$1,25\text{-}OH_2$ / $25\text{-}OH$	No
Faupel-Badger[57]	2007	Finland	50–69	296	Approximately 50	$25\text{-}OH$	No
Ahn[39]	2008	US Caucasians	67.8 (mean)	749	<15	$25\text{-}OH$	No[d]
Travis[58]	2009	Europe	61 (mean)	652	Approximately 25	$25\text{-}OH$	No
Barnett[59]	2010	United States	>65	297	24	$25\text{-}OH$	No

a Defined as ≤20 ng/mL.
b Nonsignificant increased risk.
c Increased risk found with high levels of 25-OH.
d Possible increased risk of aggressive cancer with higher 25-OH levels.

These studies may not have had a sufficient number of high-grade aggressive cancers to demonstrate a correlation between low vitamin D status and increased aggressive cancer.

Genetic Variations in VDR

Perhaps the serum level of vitamin D is not the only factor that contributes to the increase or decrease in antineoplastic activity by the VDR. Multiple studies have examined genetic polymorphisms and single nucleotide polymorphisms (SNPs) in the VDR and their relation to prostate cancer risk. A recent study[40] showed a trend to association of risk of recurrence and progression of prostate cancer with certain SNPs in the VDR and CYP27A1 (encodes 1α-hydroxylase) and CYP24A1 (encodes vitamin D–inactivating 24-hydroxylase) genes. However, these associations were not significant when corrected for multiple comparisons. Further, Mikhak and colleagues[41] analyzed multiple VDR polymorphisms along with vitamin D levels and did not show an association between common VDR polymorphisms, vitamin D levels, and prostate cancer risk.

THERAPEUTIC APPLICATIONS OF VITAMIN D IN PROSTATE CANCER

Based on preclinical studies suggesting that VDR activation enhances the activity of antineoplastic agents, studies combining therapeutic vitamin D compounds with chemotherapy have been performed. Multiple phase II studies with calcitriol in combination with various chemotherapies showed a decrease in prostate-specific antigen levels.[42–47] Specifically, the Androgen-Independent Prostate Cancer Study of Calcitriol Enhancing Taxotere (ASCENT)[42] showed an improved survival with DN-101 (a novel formulation of calcitriol designed for high-dose intermittent dosing, an approach that allows very high $1,25\text{-OH}_2$ vitamin D levels to be achieved without clinically important hypercalcemia) in combination with docetaxel weekly chemotherapy. However, the phase III development of DN-101 (ASCENT-2) was stopped early because of excess deaths in the experimental weekly docetaxel plus DN-101 arm versus the standard arm of every 3-week docetaxel plus prednisone. The difference in docetaxel regimens may explain some of the differences in this study; however, after the results of ASCENT-2 were revealed, the development of DN-101 was halted. Other approaches to testing high-dose intermittent VDR ligands are under way. A more targeted approach that seeks to deploy a vitamin D–based therapeutic strategy, only in patients with demonstrated vitamin D addiction at the level of their

tumor, may uncover clinical benefits that are not detectable in unselected populations.

SUMMARY

Overall there is compelling biologic evidence for vitamin D's role in prostate cancer development and progression; however, the clinical data have not consistently demonstrated a link. The aforementioned limits of the case-control and case-cohort studies may be the reason that there is no compelling clinical demonstration of the association between low vitamin D levels and increased prostate cancer risk; however, the absence of a clinically significant link needs to be considered. There are still important questions in this field that need to be answered, including if local prostate production of active $1,25\text{-OH}_2$ vitamin D is an important factor in prostate cancer pathogenesis, can measured local prostate vitamin D status correlate more closely with prostate cancer risk, and, if so, how this is impacted by vitamin D supplementation or treatment. In addition, studies that examine more aggressive vitamin D supplementation and prostate cancer risk are of interest.

The recent IOM recommendations for daily vitamin D supplementation need to be interpreted in the context of the data that are available to the institute. These recommendations have come about through analysis of the current medical literature, and because there are no good long-term studies with higher-dose vitamin D supplementation, there can be no consensus recommendation for the average person to take more than 600 IU of vitamin D per day.

At present, there are no consistent data to support high dose vitamin D supplementation for the average patient with prostate cancer for the treatment or halting of cancer progression. In addition, there are no data to support therapeutic use of vitamin D and its analogs in treating prostate cancer. Additional studies are needed to determine if higher doses of vitamin D supplements could benefit selected populations (ie, the elderly or patients with cancer) even if they may not be beneficial for the general population addressed by the IOM report. At present, according to the National Institutes of Health, there are multiple ongoing studies involving higher doses of vitamin D, up to 5000 IU per day, with an average supplementation of approximately 2000 IU per day. Most studies are for noncancer diagnoses or healthy patients, but once the results of these higher supplementation studies are known, there will perhaps be a consensus on whether higher doses of vitamin D are beneficial. For the average patient with prostate cancer, a recommended minimum supplementation of 600 IU of vitamin D per day, with testing at baseline to determine if additional supplementation is needed for deficiency levels (<20 ng/mL), is reasonable.

REFERENCES

1. Schwartz GG, Hulka BS. Is vitamin D deficiency a risk factor for prostate cancer? (Hypothesis). Anticancer Res 1990;10(5A):1307–11.
2. Hanchette CL, Schwartz GG. Geographic patterns of prostate cancer mortality. Evidence for a protective effect of ultraviolet radiation. Cancer 1992;70(12):2861–9.
3. Luscombe CJ, Fryer AA, French ME, et al. Exposure to ultraviolet radiation: association with susceptibility and age at presentation with prostate cancer. Lancet 2001;358(9282):641–2.
4. Grant WB. An estimate of premature cancer mortality in the U.S. due to inadequate doses of solar ultraviolet-B radiation. Cancer 2002;94(6):1867–75.
5. Bodiwala D, Luscombe CJ, French ME, et al. Susceptibility to prostate cancer: studies on interactions between UVR exposure and skin type. Carcinogenesis 2003;24(4):711–7.
6. John EM, Schwartz GG, Koo J, et al. Sun exposure, vitamin D receptor gene polymorphisms, and risk of advanced prostate cancer. Cancer Res 2005;65(12):5470–9.
7. Schwartz GG, Hanchette CL. UV, latitude, and spatial trends in prostate cancer mortality: all sunlight is not the same (United States). Cancer Causes Control 2006;17(8):1091–101.
8. Chen TC, Wang L, Whitlatch LW, et al. Prostatic 25-hydroxyvitamin D-1alpha-hydroxylase and its implication in prostate cancer. J Cell Biochem 2003;88(2):315–22.
9. Schwartz GG, Whitlatch LW, Chen TC, et al. Human prostate cells synthesize 1,25-dihydroxyvitamin D3 from 25-hydroxyvitamin D3. Cancer Epidemiol Biomarkers Prev 1998;7(5):391–5.
10. Nanes MS, Kuno H, Demay MB, et al. A single upstream element confers responsiveness to 1,25-dihydroxyvitamin D3 and tumor necrosis factor-alpha in the rat osteocalcin gene. Endocrinology 1994;134(3):1113–20.
11. Liu M, Lee MH, Cohen M, et al. Transcriptional activation of the Cdk inhibitor p21 by vitamin D3 leads to the induced differentiation of the myelomonocytic cell line U937. Genes Dev 1996;10(2):142–53.
12. Guzey M, Kitada S, Reed JC. Apoptosis induction by 1alpha,25-dihydroxyvitamin D3 in prostate cancer. Mol Cancer Ther 2002;1(9):667–77.
13. Peng L, Malloy PJ, Feldman D. Identification of a functional vitamin D response element in the human insulin-like growth factor binding protein-3 promoter. Mol Endocrinol 2004;18(5):1109–19.
14. Hakim I, Bar-Shavit Z. Modulation of TNF-alpha expression in bone marrow macrophages: involvement of vitamin D response element. J Cell Biochem 2003;88(5):986–98.
15. McGaffin KR, Chrysogelos SA. Identification and characterization of a response element in the EGFR promoter that mediates transcriptional repression by 1,25-dihydroxyvitamin D3 in breast cancer cells. J Mol Endocrinol 2005;35(1):117–33.
16. Zhuang SH, Burnstein KL. Antiproliferative effect of 1alpha,25-dihydroxyvitamin D3 in human prostate cancer cell line LNCaP involves reduction of cyclin-dependent kinase 2 activity and persistent G1 accumulation. Endocrinology 1998;139(3):1197–207.
17. Miller GJ, Stapleton GE, Ferrara JA, et al. The human prostatic carcinoma cell line LNCaP expresses biologically active, specific receptors for 1 alpha,25-dihydroxyvitamin D3. Cancer Res 1992;52(3):515–20.
18. Skowronski RJ, Peehl DM, Feldman D. Vitamin D and prostate cancer: 1,25 dihydroxyvitamin D3 receptors and actions in human prostate cancer cell lines. Endocrinology 1993;132(5):1952–60.
19. Peehl DM, Skowronski RJ, Leung GK, et al. Antiproliferative effects of 1,25-dihydroxyvitamin D3 on primary cultures of human prostatic cells. Cancer Res 1994;54(3):805–10.
20. Oades GM, Dredge K, Kirby RS, et al. Vitamin D receptor-dependent antitumour effects of 1,25-dihydroxyvitamin D3 and two synthetic analogues in three in vivo models of prostate cancer. BJU Int 2002;90(6):607–16.
21. Hsu JY, Feldman D, McNeal JE, et al. Reduced 1alpha-hydroxylase activity in human prostate cancer cells correlates with decreased susceptibility to 25-hydroxyvitamin D3-induced growth inhibition. Cancer Res 2001;61(7):2852–6.
22. Whitlatch LW, Young MV, Schwartz GG, et al. 25-Hydroxyvitamin D-1alpha-hydroxylase activity is diminished in human prostate cancer cells and is enhanced by gene transfer. J Steroid Biochem Mol Biol 2002;81(2):135–40.
23. Robsahm TE, Tretli S, Dahlback A, et al. Vitamin D3 from sunlight may improve the prognosis of breast-, colon- and prostate cancer (Norway). Cancer Causes Control 2004;15(2):149–58.
24. Lagunova Z, Porojnicu AC, Dahlback A, et al. Prostate cancer survival is dependent on season of diagnosis. Prostate 2007;67(12):1362–70.
25. Ahn J, Albanes D, Peters U, et al. Dairy products, calcium intake, and risk of prostate cancer in the prostate, lung, colorectal, and ovarian cancer screening trial. Cancer Epidemiol Biomarkers Prev 2007;16(12):2623–30.
26. Rodriguez C, McCullough ML, Mondul AM, et al. Calcium, dairy products, and risk of prostate cancer in a prospective cohort of United States men. Cancer Epidemiol Biomarkers Prev 2003;12(7):597–603.

27. Park Y, Mitrou PN, Kipnis V, et al. Calcium, dairy foods, and risk of incident and fatal prostate cancer: the NIH-AARP Diet and Health Study. Am J Epidemiol 2007;166(11):1270–9.

28. Chan JM, Pietinen P, Virtanen M, et al. Diet and prostate cancer risk in a cohort of smokers, with a specific focus on calcium and phosphorus (Finland). Cancer Causes Control 2000;11(9):859–67.

29. Baron JA, Beach M, Wallace K, et al. Risk of prostate cancer in a randomized clinical trial of calcium supplementation. Cancer Epidemiol Biomarkers Prev 2005;14(3):586–9.

30. Berndt SI, Carter HB, Landis PK, et al. Calcium intake and prostate cancer risk in a long-term aging study: the Baltimore Longitudinal Study of Aging. Urology 2002;60(6):1118–23.

31. Tavani A, Gallus S, Franceschi S, et al. Calcium, dairy products, and the risk of prostate cancer. Prostate 2001;48(2):118–21.

32. Tavani A, Bertuccio P, Bosetti C, et al. Dietary intake of calcium, vitamin D, phosphorus and the risk of prostate cancer. Eur Urol 2005;48(1):27–33.

33. Kristal AR, Arnold KB, Neuhouser ML, et al. Diet, supplement use, and prostate cancer risk: results from the prostate cancer prevention trial. Am J Epidemiol 2010;172(5):566–77.

34. Kristal AR, Cohen JH, Qu P, et al. Associations of energy, fat, calcium, and vitamin D with prostate cancer risk. Cancer Epidemiol Biomarkers Prev 2002;11(8):719–25.

35. Chan JM, Giovannucci E, Andersson SO, et al. Dairy products, calcium, phosphorous, vitamin D, and risk of prostate cancer (Sweden). Cancer Causes Control 1998;9(6):559–66.

36. Giovannucci E, Liu Y, Rimm EB, et al. Prospective study of predictors of vitamin D status and cancer incidence and mortality in men. J Natl Cancer Inst 2006;98(7):451–9.

37. Skinner HG, Schwartz GG. Serum calcium and incident and fatal prostate cancer in the National Health and Nutrition Examination Survey. Cancer Epidemiol Biomarkers Prev 2008;17(9):2302–5.

38. Tuohimaa P, Tenkanen L, Ahonen M, et al. Both high and low levels of blood vitamin D are associated with a higher prostate cancer risk: a longitudinal, nested case-control study in the Nordic countries. Int J Cancer 2004;108(1):104–8.

39. Ahn J, Peters U, Albanes D, et al. Serum vitamin D concentration and prostate cancer risk: a nested case-control study. J Natl Cancer Inst 2008;100(11):796–804.

40. Holt SK, Kwon EM, Koopmeiners JS, et al. Vitamin D pathway gene variants and prostate cancer prognosis. Prostate 2010;70(13):1448–60.

41. Mikhak B, Hunter DJ, Spiegelman D, et al. Vitamin D receptor (VDR) gene polymorphisms and haplotypes, interactions with plasma 25-hydroxyvitamin D and 1,25-dihydroxyvitamin D, and prostate cancer risk. Prostate 2007;67(9):911–23.

42. Beer TM, Ryan CW, Venner PM, et al. Double-blinded randomized study of high-dose calcitriol plus docetaxel compared with placebo plus docetaxel in androgen-independent prostate cancer: a report from the ASCENT Investigators. J Clin Oncol 2007;25(6):669–74.

43. Beer TM, Eilers KM, Garzotto M, et al. Weekly high-dose calcitriol and docetaxel in metastatic androgen-independent prostate cancer. J Clin Oncol 2003;21(1):123–8.

44. Beer TM, Garzotto M, Katovic NM. High-dose calcitriol and carboplatin in metastatic androgen-independent prostate cancer. Am J Clin Oncol 2004;27(5):535–41.

45. Tiffany NM, Ryan CW, Garzotto M, et al. High dose pulse calcitriol, docetaxel and estramustine for androgen independent prostate cancer: a phase I/II study. J Urol 2005;174(3):888–92.

46. Trump DL, Potter DM, Muindi J, et al. Phase II trial of high-dose, intermittent calcitriol (1,25 dihydroxyvitamin D3) and dexamethasone in androgen-independent prostate cancer. Cancer 2006;106(10):2136–42.

47. Chan JS, Beer TM, Quinn DI, et al. A phase II study of high-dose calcitriol combined with mitoxantrone and prednisone for androgen-independent prostate cancer. BJU Int 2008;102(11):1601–6.

48. Giovannucci E, Rimm EB, Wolk A, et al. Calcium and fructose intake in relation to risk of prostate cancer. Cancer Res 1998;58(3):442–7.

49. Corder EH, Guess HA, Hulka BS, et al. Vitamin D and prostate cancer: a prediagnostic study with stored sera. Cancer Epidemiol Biomarkers Prev 1993;2(5):467–72.

50. Ahonen MH, Tenkanen L, Teppo L, et al. Prostate cancer risk and prediagnostic serum 25-hydroxyvitamin D levels (Finland). Cancer Causes Control 2000;11(9):847–52.

51. Li H, Stampfer MJ, Hollis JB, et al. A prospective study of plasma vitamin D metabolites, vitamin D receptor polymorphisms, and prostate cancer. PLoS Med 2007;4(3):e103.

52. Braun MM, Helzlsouer KJ, Hollis BW, et al. Prostate cancer and prediagnostic levels of serum vitamin D metabolites (Maryland, United States). Cancer Causes Control 1995;6(3):235–9.

53. Gann PH, Hennekens CH, Hollis BW, et al. Circulating vitamin D metabolites in relation to subsequent development of prostate cancer. Cancer Epidemiol Biomarkers Prev 1996;5(2):121–6.

54. Nomura AM, Stemmermann GN, Lee J, et al. Serum vitamin D metabolite levels and the subsequent development of prostate cancer (Hawaii, United States). Cancer Causes Control 1998;9(4):425–32.

55. Platz EA, Leitzmann MF, Hollis BW, et al. Plasma 1,25-dihydroxy- and 25-hydroxyvitamin D and subsequent risk of prostate cancer. Cancer Causes Control 2004;15(3):255–65.

56. Jacobs ET, Giuliano AR, Martínez ME, et al. Plasma levels of 25-hydroxyvitamin D, 1,25-dihydroxyvitamin D and the risk of prostate cancer. J Steroid Biochem Mol Biol 2004;89–90(1–5):533–7.

57. Faupel-Badger JM, Diaw L, Albanes D, et al. Lack of association between serum levels of 25-hydroxyvitamin D and the subsequent risk of prostate cancer in Finnish men. Cancer Epidemiol Biomarkers Prev 2007;16(12):2784–6.

58. Travis RC, Crowe FL, Allen NE, et al. Serum vitamin D and risk of prostate cancer in a case-control analysis nested within the European Prospective Investigation into Cancer and Nutrition (EPIC). Am J Epidemiol 2009;169(10):1223–32.

59. Barnett CM, Nielson CM, Shannon J, et al. Serum 25-OH vitamin D levels and risk of developing prostate cancer in older men. Cancer Causes Control 2010;21(8):1297–303.

Prostate Imaging Modalities that Can Be Used for Complementary and Alternative Medicine Clinical Studies

Reginald W. Dusing, MD[a],*, Jeanne A. Drisko, MD[b],
Gordon G. Grado, MD[c,d], Mark Levine, MD[e],
Jeffrey M. Holzbeierlein, MD[f], Peter Van Veldhuizen, MD[g]

KEYWORDS

- Prostate cancer • Bone scan • TRUS • PET • ProstaScint
- SPECT • C-11 acetate • Vitamin C

THE PROBLEM

Prostate cancer is the most common type of cancer found in American men other than skin cancer and is the second leading cause of cancer death among men—second only to lung cancer. For 2010, the American Cancer Society estimated that there were approximately 220,000 new cases of prostate cancer diagnosed in the United States and approximately 32,000 men died of the disease. These statistics suggest that 1 in 6 men will be diagnosed with prostate cancer during their lifetime (1 in 5 for African American men) and 1 in 36 will die of this disease—statistics that are strikingly similar to breast cancer statistics for women.[1] Alarmingly, the general population is unaware of these risks because men are reluctant to talk about their disease or go for annual examinations. In many ways, men still have a denial mindset similar to the mindset women had toward breast cancer before former First Lady Betty Ford's efforts to destigmatize breast cancer. In 1978, Mrs. Ford publicly acknowledged her breast cancer diagnosis and subsequent mastectomy. Her declaration of her

Dr Reginald Dusing's work was supported by The Clinical Radiology Foundation and the Molecular Imaging Research Fund of the KU Endowment foundation of the University of Kansas. Dr Mark Levine was supported by the intramural research program, National Institute of Diabetes, Digestive, and Kidney Diseases, National Institutes of Health.

Financial disclosures: the authors have no conflicts of interest to report.

[a] Division of Nuclear Medicine, Department of Radiology, Kansas University Medical Center, MS 4032, 3901 Rainbow Boulevard, Kansas City, KS 66160-7234, USA
[b] Program in Integrative Medicine, University of Kansas Medical Center, 3901 Rainbow Boulevard, Kansas City, KS 66160, USA
[c] Southwest Oncology Centers, 2926 North Civic Center Plaza, Scottsdale, AZ 85251, USA
[d] Department of Radiation Oncology, University of Minnesota, Minneapolis, MN, USA
[e] Molecular and Clinical Nutrition Section, National Institutes of Health, Building 10, Room 4D52, MSC 1372, Bethesda, MD 20892-1372, USA
[f] Prostate Cancer Prevention Program, Department of Urology Surgery, University of Kansas Medical Center, 3901 Rainbow Boulevard, Kansas City, KS 66160, USA
[g] Division of Hematology and Oncology, Department of Internal Medicine, University of Kansas Medical Center, 3901 Rainbow Boulevard, Kansas City, KS 66160, USA
* Corresponding author.
E-mail address: rdusing@kumc.edu

Urol Clin N Am 38 (2011) 343–357
doi:10.1016/j.ucl.2011.04.003
0094-0143/11/$ – see front matter

diagnosis and ensuing determination to publicly fight breast cancer encouraged early detection and inspired thousands of American women who were also coping with the disease. American men have not had a similar advocate for prostate cancer step forward and raise public awareness to this same level. This unfortunate disparity in awareness is reinforced by disparate levels of funding for breast cancer and prostate cancer at the National Institutes of Health. In 2010, $824 million was dedicated to breast cancer research whereas less than half that amount—$362 million—was dedicated to prostate cancer research.[2]

Aside from these public health concerns, the problem is compounded by the elusiveness of diagnosis and localization. Early prostate cancer usually has no symptoms. Prostate-specific antigen (PSA) screening can usually detect prostate cancer years earlier than it would be detected by a digital rectal examination or the development of symptoms. Although there is no absolute cutoff between a normal and an abnormal PSA level, screening programs in the United States have commonly used greater than 4 ng/mL to define a positive test. PSA screening, however, has several limitations. Many men who do not have prostate cancer screen PSA positive, whereas some men with biopsy-proved prostate cancer do not have elevated PSA levels. To evaluate the efficacy of screening the at-risk male population, 2 large randomized trials of prostate cancer screening with PSA testing have been completed. The results are conflicting. The United States–based Prostate, Lung, Colorectal, and Ovarian Cancer Screening Trial did not observe a correlation between screening and decreased prostate cancer mortality, whereas the European Randomized Study of Screening for Prostate Cancer demonstrated a 20% reduction in prostate cancer mortality among men who were screened for PSA compared with those who were not screened for PSA.[1,3,4]

Whether the diagnosis of prostate cancer is suggested by elevation of PSA or by physical findings on digital rectal examination, the initial diagnosis is confirmed by biopsy, often guided by transrectal ultrasound (TRUS). Of the 220,000 new cases diagnosed in 2010, approximately 75%, or 165,000 patients, will choose to have potentially curative therapy—radical prostatectomy or radiation therapy.[1] Unfortunately, these therapies will fail in approximately 40% of these 165,000 patients, or approximately 66,000 men, in whom PSA levels will rise in the following years, indicating recurrence of tumor.[1] The challenge then is to localize the recurrence at an early stage to try to arrest the disease with radiation therapy or surgery (salvage therapy) to possibly effect a cure rather than simply relegate patients to palliative hormonal therapy, which is expensive, carries significant side effects, and ultimately fails in almost all cases.

Many different imaging modalities have been used with varying success to try to localize sites of recurrence (**Fig. 1**). Most commonly, patients with a rising PSA undergo CT imaging of the abdomen and pelvis along with a radionuclide bone scan. Ultrasound, MRI, indium 111 (^{111}In) capromab pendetide (ProstaScint) single-photon emission computed tomography (SPECT), fluorodeoxyglucose F 18 positron emission tomography ([^{18}F]FDG-PET or FDG-PET), and carbon 11 acetate PET ([^{11}C]acetate-PET) or [^{18}F]choline-PET, however, can be used effectively to help localize recurrence in various clinical presentations. This article provides a brief overview of each imaging modality and its potential applications and limitations.

BONE SCAN

Bone scanning has been used to look for osseous metastases in prostate cancer since the introduction of the modern Anger gamma camera to nuclear medicine in the 1960s. Bone scans are more sensitive for detecting osteoblastic metastasis than are planar radiographs because 30% of the bone matrix must be affected for metastases to be detectable by conventional radiography. Studies dating back to 1976 have shown that at least 62% of patients with a positive bone scan have normal planar radiographs.[5] Bisphosphonates are labeled with radioactive technetium Tc 99m (^{99m}Tc) to make a radiopharmaceutical (^{99m}Tc–methylene diphosphonate) that is injected intravenously. The radiopharmaceutical binds to the bony matrix of the skeleton over a period of 3 to 6 hours, accumulating at sites of osteoblastic activity. Patients are then scanned from the vertex of the skull to the knees or below to identify sites of abnormal accumulation that suggest metastases. Characteristically, the frequency of metastases to any given bone is proportional to the amount of red marrow that bone contains, and, as a general rule in prostate cancer, metastases occur in the axial skeleton before they occur in the appendicular skeleton. Correlating bone scans with recent planar radiographs or CT is often helpful to distinguish osteophytes or previous trauma from metastases. Nevertheless, the yield of positive findings in bone scans is low in men with early-stage increases in PSA levels. Conventional bone scanning is rarely positive when PSA levels are less than 10.0 ng/mL and remains fairly insensitive when the PSA levels are less than 20.0 ng/mL.[6–9] In a study at the Mayo Clinic of 306 prostate cancer patients with a serum PSA level of 20 ng/mL or less, Chybowski

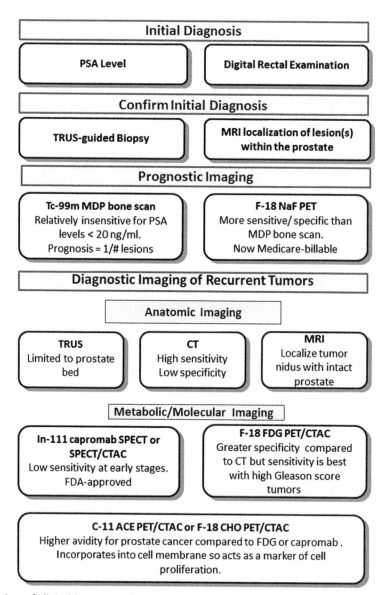

Fig. 1. An overview of clinical imaging techniques that are applied to diagnosis of prostate cancer.

and colleagues[10] found that only 1 patient, who had a PSA of 18.2 ng/mL, had a positive bone scan. Nevertheless, a conventional radionuclide bone scan is a valuable prognostic indicator in patients with advanced disease because prostate cancer patients with a positive bone scan are known to have a shortened lifespan (**Fig. 2**).[11]

Additionally, several studies suggest that [18F] sodium fluoride–PET bone scanning is more sensitive and more specific than ^{99m}Tc–methylene diphosphonate bone scanning in identifying osteoblastic metastases in most cancers and may be up to 100% sensitive and specific with 100% positive predictive values and negative predictive values in prostate cancer patients with PSA levels greater

than 20 ng/mL.[12,13] In February 2011, the National Oncologic PET Registry added [18F]sodium fluoride–PET bone scanning as a Medicare-billable diagnostic option for evaluating osseous metastatic lesions for all cancers. The medical literature to date contains no information, however, on the PSA value that correlates with a positive sodium fluoride PET bone scan, and the clinical significance of such a threshold remains to be determined.

ULTRASOUND

Ultrasound has long been used to detect prostate cancer. In the late 1980s and early 1990s, there was great hope among many of those in the

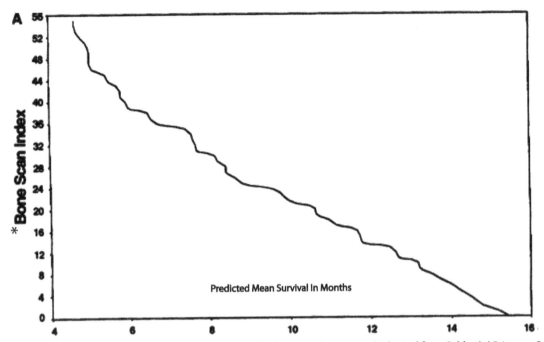

Fig. 2. *Bone scan index = 0.92 × the total number of lesions on a bone scan. (Adapted from Sabbatini P, Larson S, Kremer A, et al. Prognostic significance of extent of disease in bone in patients with androgen-independent prostate cancer. J Clin Oncol 1999;17(3):948–57; with permission.)*

imaging community that, with the development of dedicated ultrasound transducers, TRUS would prove useful for screening. Such was not the case. The findings on TRUS are not sufficiently specific to make it a cost-effective tool for screening the general population. Currently, in addition to guiding biopsies of nodules detected on digital rectal examination for the initial diagnosis of prostate cancer, TRUS is used in looking for recurrence in the prostate bed after radical prostatectomy with subsequent biochemical recurrence heralded by rising PSA levels. Beyond the prostate bed, however, ultrasound lacks sufficient tissue penetration to be of use in looking for pelvic nodes or more distant metastases.[14,15]

CT

Because CT renders precise anatomic images, it has become the mainstay of advanced imaging in most medical institutions. Although the average CT scanner in most communities today can easily resolve anatomic detail as small as the ossicles of the middle ear, the issue in prostate cancer imaging is specificity not sensitivity.[16,17] The question is, "What does the finding of a 1-cm lymph node localized in the pelvis of a patient with a rising PSA level suggest?" Does this finding confirm recurrent prostate cancer? Does the finding mean that the node contains metastatic tissue? It may

simply be a prominent normal node or perhaps a node enlarged in reaction to infection or inflammation elsewhere in that node's lymphatic drainage area. Since CT's inception, radiologists have relied on size criteria—if a node is less than 1 cm, it is benign; if it is more than 1 cm, it is pathologic. Not only is this intuitively illogical because a node must contain a critical mass of metastatic cells before it starts to enlarge but also, statistically, these criteria have been shown to provide less than ideal specificity for diagnosis. A vivid illustration of this is the case of lung cancer. In 2000, even before the advent of the current PET scanners that are coupled to low-dose CT for attenuation correction (PET/CTAC), Pieterman and colleagues[18] showed, in a sample of more than 100 lung cancer patients, that the specificity for detection of mediastinal metastases with FDG-PET was 86% but the specificity for detection with CT was only 66%. This introduces the case for functional molecular imaging over anatomic imaging (discussed later). First MRI is discussed, which is in many ways a hybrid of anatomic and physiologic imaging.

MRI

Because of its unique ability to characterize the content and distribution of water in various tissues of the body and its good anatomic resolution, MRI has shown great promise for the detection of both the primary lesion and metastasis in prostate cancer. It is an excellent technique for localizing the nidus of tumor in the intact prostate gland and can be used in presurgical planning to see whether the tumor has spread beyond the confines of the prostate capsule or has invaded the neurovascular bundle.[19] It has also shown usefulness in anatomically identifying metastatic nodes in the pelvis.[16,20] Issues of specificity remain unsolved, however. Groundbreaking research in the Netherlands using a ferromagnetic contrast agent with MRI holds promise for improving specificity of diagnosis in finding nodal metastases, but this technique is years away from possible Food and Drug Administration (FDA) approval or Centers for Medicare and Medicaid Services reimbursement certification.[21] Additionally, MRI has been of limited use in finding distant metastases, because, by the nature of the technology, each region of the body needs to be scanned separately, adding to the expense and length of scanning time.

CAPROMAB PENDETIDE SPECT OR SPECT/CTAC

First introduced in the late 1990s, capromab is a hamster monoclonal antibody that selectively binds to prostate-specific membrane antigen, a surface biomarker that is present on human prostate cancer cells at various stages but is not present on normal cells. Labeled with ^{111}In, the antibody is injected into a patient, with SPECT or SPECT/CTAC imaging performed 4 to 6 days later. Although elegant in theory—using an imaging isotope labeled to an antibody that is targeted specifically for prostate cancer cells, in practice the results have been less than stellar. The scans can appear murky, making them difficult to read and the interpretation learning curve for nuclear radiologists is steep. Moreover, correlating capromab scan findings with actual pathologic findings has not always yielded reassuring results. For example, in a prospective, preoperative study with tissue confirmation, Ponsky and colleagues[22] at the Cleveland Clinic found a sensitivity of only 17% and a positive predictive value of only 11% and concluded a high false-positive rate and a low positive predictive value overestimated metastatic lymph node disease. As a result of these difficulties with scan interpretation, many urologists and oncologists have become disillusioned with the examination.

PET/CTAC

Given the limitations of anatomic imaging (described previously), is there any hope for a breakthrough in imaging prostate cancer, especially metastatic or recurrent prostate cancer? The answer may be within the realm of functional molecular imaging, specifically PET coregistered with low-dose CTAC, which gives both metabolic and molecular information on a cellular level coupled with anatomic definition. As discussed previously, FDG-PET has shown a greater specificity compared with anatomic imaging in the staging and management of lung cancer. The differences in sensitivity and specificity for FDG-PET versus CT in the diagnosis, staging, and detecting recurrence in lung cancer have been shown in some series to result in a change in patient management 37% of the time.[11] For colorectal cancer recurrence, change in management is seen in 31% of the patients, with similar advantages seen in lymphoma, melanoma, and breast cancer. Most common cancers—lung, lymphoma, melanoma, colorectal, head and neck, esophageal, transitional cell, and breast—have increased metabolic needs to grow rapidly and proliferate. The basic metabolic substrate for these tumor cells is glucose. To meet the increased need for glucose, these tumor cells have increased glucose transport mechanisms and are thus considered glucose avid. FDG is made by chemically substituting cyclotron-produced radioactive ^{18}F for a hydroxyl group on the hexose ring of glucose. The resulting compound, FDG, after being phosphorylated, is transported through the cell membrane in the same manner as glucose. The key metabolic difference between glucose and FDG is that FDG is not as easily dephosphorylated and then metabolized by tumor cells as glucose. Therefore, by virtue of its increased transport into the cell and decreased metabolism within the cell, FDG accumulates to a greater extent in tumor cells than surrounding normal tissue. This makes the radioactive signal of the FDG in the tumor cells more conspicuous than the signal from any normal cells that may have also taken up FDG, thus rendering tumors easier to localize than by CT alone. In addition, it allows differentiating metabolically active tumor from scar tissue after therapy.

Unfortunately for prostate cancer patients, prostate cancer cells are not particularly glucose avid, except in more aggressive cell lines, such as those with high Gleason scores. The reason for this is unclear. Some investigators have postulated that because prostate cancer can be more indolent, perhaps it does not have high glucose requirements. This simplistic explanation is contradicted, however, by the fact that another genitourinary tumor, renal cell carcinoma, is highly aggressive yet is also not highly glucose avid. So, the answer must lie in prostate cancer metabolism on a cellular level. The good news is that other compounds that are ubiquitous in the body, acetate and choline, have a unique metabolism in prostate cancer. These compounds are used in the synthesis of the phospholipid bilayer of the cell membrane. In normal prostate cells, acetate is metabolized through the Krebs cycle for energy. With the increased cellular proliferation of prostate cancer, however, acetate is used for cell membrane synthesis.[23] By substituting cyclotron-produced ^{11}C into the acetate molecule for a nonradioactive carbon 12 atom, ^{11}C]acetate is able to be detected incorporated into the cell membranes of proliferating prostate cancer by means of PET/CTAC.

Data from both the United States and Europe have shown similar results detecting recurrent prostate cancer with either ^{11}C]acetate or [18F] choline. From a practical point of view, [18F]choline is easier to ship from the cyclotron to the PET scan site because ^{18}F has a 110-minute half-life compared with the 20-minute half-life of ^{11}C, which generally limits ^{11}C]acetate use to PET scanners within close proximity of a cyclotron. Alternatively, ^{11}C]acetate has little urinary tract excretion whereas [18F]choline has significant urinary excretion that can potentially obscure recurrent tumors in the prostate bed and along the course of the ureters. Finally, in the United States, [18F]choline is not FDA approved, whereas ^{11}C]acetate has been in the United States Pharmacopeia for more than 20 years with a great patient safety record in cardiac PET imaging. Since the first article in the medical literature describing the utility of ^{11}C] acetate in imaging prostate cancer by Oyama and colleagues[24] in 2002, there have been more than 50 refereed journal articles in the world literature describing the application of ^{11}C]acetate and [18F]choline-PET in prostate cancer. Since 2002, however, most of the ^{11}C]acetate and [18F]choline clinical PET prostate studies have been performed in Europe, because difficulties in getting FDA approval and CMS reimbursement are not an issue in Europe as they have been in the United States.

In 1998, Haseman[25] published a comparison of capromab SPECT versus FDG-PET and found capromab superior. In 2003, Oyama and colleagues[26] compared ^{11}C]acetate-PET to FDG-PET in 46 patients and found ^{11}C]acetate to have a putative sensitivity of 59% versus 17% for FDG-PET. The third leg of the metaphorical triangle would be to compare capromab SPECT to ^{11}C]acetate-PET, but to date there have been no published data comparing the 2 studies. However, between February 22, 2007 and February 21, 2008, in the Department of Radiology, Division of Nuclear Medicine at the University of Kansas Hospital, Kansas City, Kansas, the authors conducted a pilot study prospectively comparing capromab SPECT to ^{11}C]acetate-PET in each of 20 men who had undergone radical prostatectomy for primary prostate cancer and experienced biochemical recurrence, defined as a rise in PSA postprostatectomy from a baseline of 0.0 ng/mL to 0.2 ng/mL or greater. Using 3 nuclear medicine subspecialty trained board certified radiologists who read all the studies in a blinded manner, the results showed that for early recurrence—an average lymph node size of 1.03 cm and a mean PSA value of 1.0—there was a putative sensitivity of 85% for ^{11}C]acetate-PET/ CTAC versus a 30% putative sensitivity for capromab SPECT.

Based on these results and findings in the world literature corroborating the high sensitivity of ^{11}C] acetate-PET/CTAC in detecting metastatic prostate cancer, the authors embarked on a program offering ^{11}C]acetate-PET scans to physician-referred patients with biochemically recurrent prostate cancer—currently defined as patients who have undergone a radical prostatectomy and who achieved a postoperative PSA value of 0.0 ng/mL that subsequently rose to greater than 0.4 ng/mL[27] or for patients who have received definitive external beam radiotherapy or brachytherapy, with recurrence defined as a PSA rise of greater than 2.0 ng/mL above the post-treatment nadir.[28] Since 2007, the authors have performed more than 200 clinical ^{11}C]acetate-PET scans at the University of Kansas Hospital, with encouraging clinical results based on outcomes. The following 3 cases serve as illustrations of the potential of functional molecular imaging.

CASE 1: A COMPARISON OF CT VERSUS ^{11}C] ACETATE-PET/CTAC IN DIAGNOSING RETROPERITONEAL LYMPHADENOPATHY SUGGESTING RECURRENT METASTATIC DISEASE IN A 73-YEAR-OLD MAN WITH RISING PSA LEVELS

Presentation

This 73-year-old man was first diagnosed with prostate cancer in April 2008. Diagnostic findings included a tumor biopsy that had a Gleason score of 7 (4 + 3). The patient subsequently was treated with brachytherapy radioactive seed implantation in May 2008. After brachytherapy, the patient's PSA levels were 0.7 ng/mL in July 2009 and 0.7 ng/mL in July 2010. By October 2010, the patient's PSA level had risen to 1.5 ng/mL, and by January 2011, the patient's PSA level was 2.2 ng/mL. Although not meeting the strict criteria for biochemical recurrence after radiation therapy, the patient and his treating physician were concerned enough to proceed with a CT scan. After an ambiguous CT report stating, "retroperitoneal lymphadenopathy concerning for metastatic disease given rising PSA," the patient was referred for a [^{11}C]acetate-PET/CTAC scan to further try identify sites of possible recurrence.

Findings

The [^{11}C]acetate-PET/CTAC transaxial images show a markedly [^{11}C]acetate-avid retroperitoneal aortocaval lymph node (pinpointed by the cross-hairs) (**Fig. 3**). Although this node did not meet the CT size criteria for a metastatic lesion (ie, not greater than 1 cm in diameter), the [^{11}C]acetate-PET/CTAC scan shows marked [^{11}C]acetate avidity suggesting this node contains metastatic prostate cancer. The middle, coronal image shows that, in addition to the primary node, the retroperitoneal lymph nodes extending in a chain caudally from the primary node are also markedly [^{11}C] acetate avid, suggesting additional metastases.

Analysis

Although CT scanning is extremely sensitive for detecting even subcentimeter lymph nodes, [^{11}C] acetate PET/CTAC provides more specificity in confirming the suspicion and location of recurrent prostate cancer.

CASE 2: A COMPARISON OF [^{111}IN] CAPROMAB-SPECT VERSUS [^{11}C]ACETATE-PET/CTAC IN DIAGNOSING SUBSEQUENT NODAL METASTASIS IN A 72-YEAR-OLD MAN WITH RISING PSA LEVELS AFTER RADICAL PROSTATECTOMY
Presentation

A 72-year-old man had undergone a radical prostatectomy in August 1999. At the time of surgery, pathology analysis of a biopsy sample showed a tumor with a Gleason score of 6 (3 + 3), with focal involvement of the capsular margin on the right side. This finding suggested that the patient had a high risk for future recurrence. On April 12, 2007, the patient's PSA level was 2.3 ng/mL. Two weeks later, the patient was evaluated by using a [^{11}C]acetate/CTAC followed immediately by [^{111}In]capromab-SPECT scan.

Findings

The [^{11}C]acetate-PET/CTAC scan shows changes consistent with radical prostatectomy, including surgical clips in the prostate bed and in the pelvic lymph node chains (**Fig. 4**). A small focus of [^{11}C] acetate-avid tissue is observed adjacent to a surgical clip on the right side of the pelvis. The

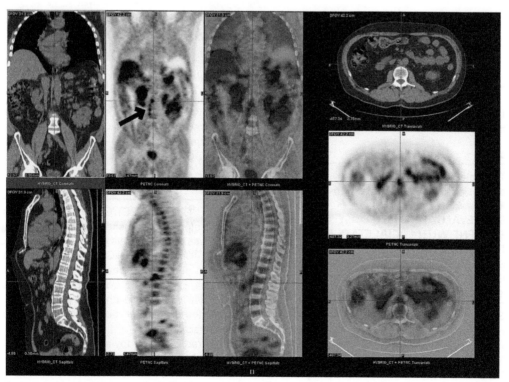

Fig. 3. Case 1. PET/CTAC images demonstrating a chain of [^{11}C]acetate-avid retroperitoneal lymph nodes (*arrow*).

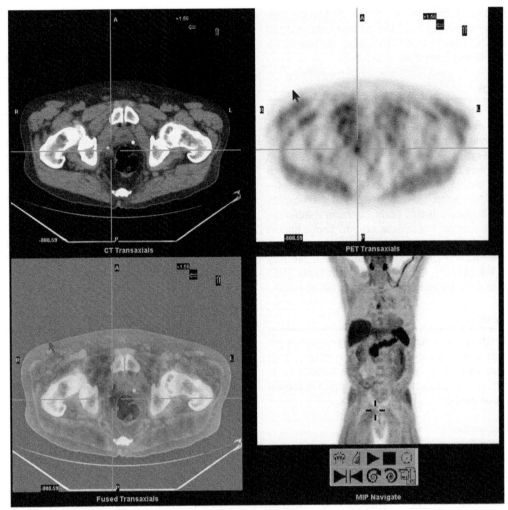

Fig. 4. Case 2. PET/CTAC images of a [^{11}C]acetate-positive pelvic lymph node recurrence adjacent to a surgical clip.

[^{111}In]capromab-SPECT can shows no evidence of capromab-avid tissue in this area (**Fig. 5**).

Analysis

[^{11}C]acetate -PET/CTAC is able to detect much smaller lesions than [^{111}In]capromab-SPECT.

CASE 3: EVALUATING RESPONSE TO TREATMENT WITH [^{11}C]ACETATE-PET/CTAC AFTER STEREOTACTIC BODY RADIATION THERAPY AND HORMONAL THERAPY IN A 53-YEAR-OLD MAN
Presentation

A 53-year-old man was first diagnosed with prostate cancer in September 2009. The tumor had a Gleason score of 8 (4 + 4) and the patient's PSA was 14 ng/mL. Eleven days after diagnosis and before therapy of any kind, a [^{11}C]acetate-PET/CTAC scan was performed. Thereafter, the patient was treated with stereotactic body radiation therapy and hormonal therapy. Therapy ended in February 2010 and a follow-up [^{11}C]acetate-PET/CTAC scan was conducted in April 2010.

Findings

Fused [^{11}C]acetate-PET/CTAC transaxial images taken before therapy show increased activity in both lobes of the prostate gland (**Fig. 6**). Additional fused [^{11}C]acetate-PET/CTAC transaxial images obtained during the same study show a focus of increased [^{11}C]acetate avidity in the left posterior iliac spine with subtle changes on CTAC in the associated trabecular bone that suggest bone metastasis (**Fig. 7**).

After radiation therapy ended in February 2010, the patient was re-evaluated, using a [^{11}C]acetate-PET/CTAC scan in April 2010. The fused [^{11}C] acetate-PET/CTAC transaxial images show marked

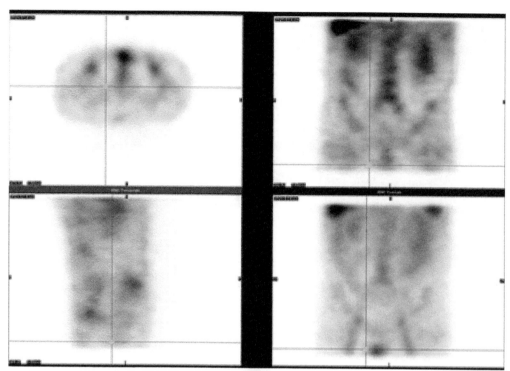

Fig. 5. Case 2. [¹¹¹In]capromab-SPECT images in 3 orthogonal planes of the same site as Fig. 4, showing no activity in a [¹¹C]acetate-positive nodal recurrence.

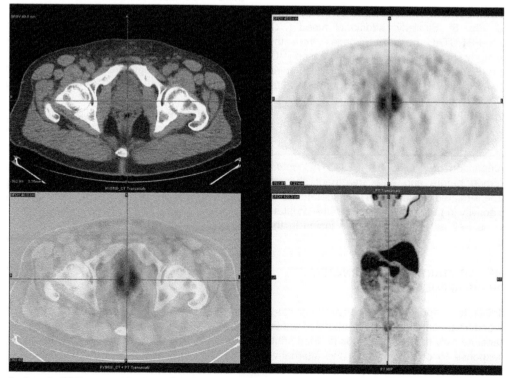

Fig. 6. Case 3. [¹¹C]acetate-PET/CTAC fused images showing elevated activity in bilateral lobes of the prostate before therapy.

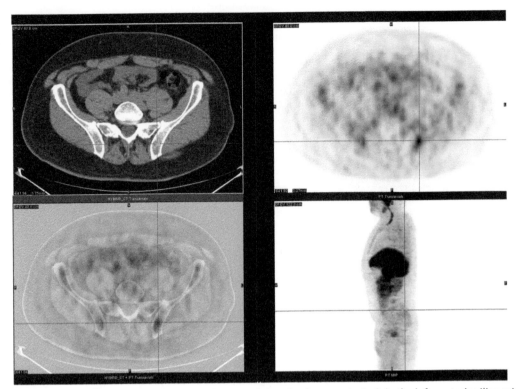

Fig. 7. Case 3. Same [^{11}C]acetate-PET/CTAC study as Fig. 6 showing bone metastasis in the left posterior iliac spine.

reduction in both the size of the ^{11}C-avid area and level of ^{11}C activity in both lobes of the prostate gland (**Fig. 8**). Similarly, additional fused [^{11}C] acetate-PET/CTAC transaxial images from the same study show that the focus of increased [^{11}C] acetate-PET avidity in the left posterior iliac spine that was observed during the September 2009 study had resolved and was no longer visible after treatment (**Fig. 9**).

Analysis

A comparison of [^{11}C]acetate-PET/CTAC scans performed before and after treatment showed treatment-related reductions in [^{11}C]acetate metabolic activity in the primary lesions in the prostate gland as well as in the metastatic lesion in the bone.

COMPLEMENTARY AND ALTERNATIVE MEDICINE APPLICATIONS

In addition to its applications in conventional diagnosis and treatment modalities in prostate cancer, [^{11}C]acetate may have applications in documenting response to complementary and alternative medicine therapies. For example, mounting evidence confirms the role of parenteral ascorbic acid as an anticancer agent.[29] Evidence shows

there is neoplastic cell death when pharmacologic ascorbate is used and the cytotoxicity is the result of hydrogen peroxide production.[30] Intravenous ascorbate has potential to benefit some patients with cancer, with minimal adverse effects.[31–33] The Program in Integrative Medicine at the Kansas University Medical Center, Kansas City, Kansas, extends these observations by reporting the following case study of one patient's dramatic response to intravenous ascorbate as a treatment for prostate cancer.

CASE 4: THE EFFECT OF HIGH DOSE INTRAVENOUS ASCORBIC ACID IN TREATING PROSTATE CANCER IN A HEALTHY 59-YEAR-OLD MAN WITH PROSTATE CANCER
Presentation

A 59-year-old man who was otherwise healthy had a rising PSA level. PSA values increased from 2.7 ng/mL in 2005 to 4.8 ng/mL in 2007. Multiple digital rectal examinations were reported to be normal. TRUS-guided biopsies in October 2007, however, revealed bilateral high-grade prostatic intraepithelial neoplasia and adenocarcinoma. The pathology slides from the biopsies were reviewed by 2 separate laboratories; both evaluations confirmed the diagnosis of prostate cancer with a Gleason score of 7 (4 + 3).

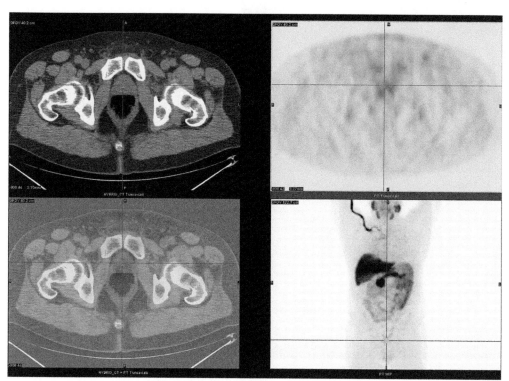

Fig. 8. Case 3. [^{11}C]acetate-PET/CTAC scan performed after external beam radiation and hormone therapy showing marked interval reduction in [^{11}C]acetate metabolism in bilateral lobes of the prostate.

The patient elected to have a radical retropubic prostatectomy, which was performed on December 19, 2007. After radical prostatectomy, pathologic evaluation of the resected tissue confirmed the diagnosis of adenocarcinoma with a Gleason score 7 (4 + 3). The tumor was confined to the right and left lobes of the prostate and there was no evidence that the tumor had extended beyond the prostate capsule. Bilateral pelvic lymphadenopathy dissection did not show evidence of lymph node invasion.

Between November 5, 2007, and December 12, 2007, after the initial biopsy results but before his surgery, the patient underwent a course of 23 intravenous ascorbic acid infusions at a maximal dose of 100-g ascorbic acid/infusion. The patient received no other therapy in the interval between biopsy and surgical resection. The patient was evaluated by using [^{11}C]acetate-PET/CTAC before and after ascorbic acid infusion.

Findings

The initial [^{11}C]acetate-PET/CTAC scan, which was conducted on November 11, 2007, before ascorbic acid infusion occurred, identified a large-volume tumor that was confined to the prostate.

(**Fig. 10**) The scan results were consistent with the subsequent postsurgical pathology stage of adenocarcinoma with a Gleason score of 7 (4 + 3). On December 14, 2007, after the last ascorbic acid infusion was completed, a [^{11}C]acetate-PET/CTAC scan was repeated before surgery. (**Fig. 11**) This scan showed a marked reduction in both the metabolic activity as determined by [^{11}C]acetate avidity and in the size of the prostate gland. When compared with the pretreatment scan, the post-treatment/presurgery scan identified a markedly decreased uptake of [^{11}C]acetate in most regions of the prostate, including those in the pretreatment biopsies that had been identified to be cancer or high-grade prostatic intraepithelial neoplasia. These observations were consistent with diminishing metabolic activity of the prostate neoplasms due to treatment with ascorbic acid infusions.

[^{11}C]acetate is an important marker of cell membrane proliferation in prostate cancer.[34] The relative metabolic activities (measured in standard uptake values [SUVs]) in both the pretreatment and post-treatment/presurgery [^{11}C]acetate-PET/CTAC scans were compared with the findings from the pathology analysis of the pretreatment

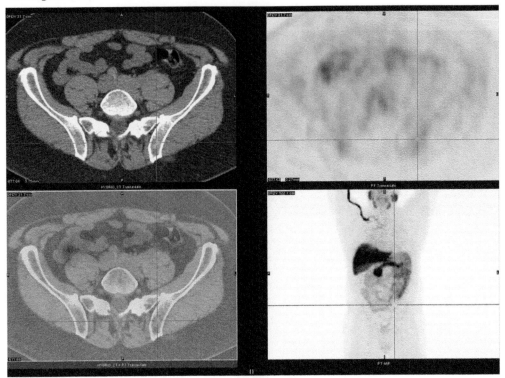

Fig. 9. Case 3. [^{11}C]acetate-PET/CTAC scan performed after external beam radiation and hormone therapy showing resolution of abnormal [^{11}C]acetate metabolism in the left iliac spine.

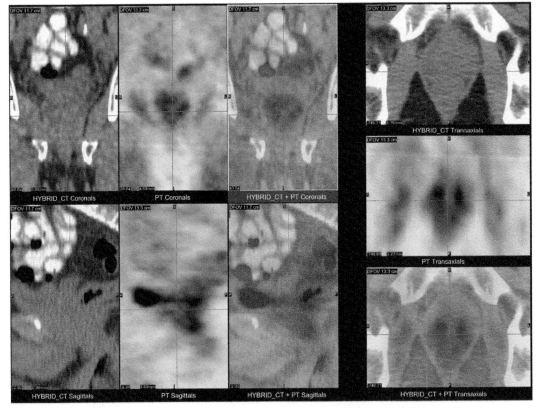

Fig. 10. Case 4. [^{11}C]acetate-PET/CTAC of the prostate gland with biopsy-proved Gleason 7 prostate cancer showing marked elevation in [^{11}C]acetate metabolism before high-dose ascorbate therapy.

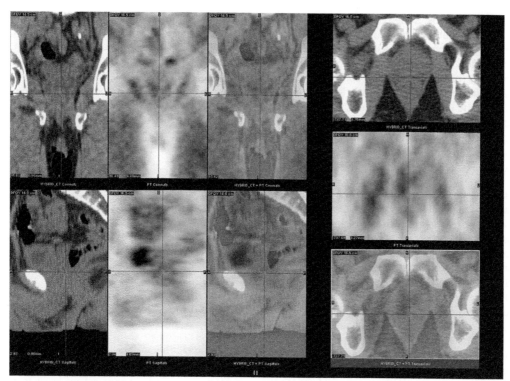

Fig. 11. Case 4. [^{11}C]acetate-PET/CTAC of same patient as Fig. 10 after 23 intravenous doses of ascorbic acid shows marked interval reduction in elevated C11 ACE metabolism.

and surgically resected tissue biopsy specimens (**Fig. 12**). Compared with the pretreatment scan, the post-treatment scan revealed that uptake of [^{11}C]acetate was reduced in all areas of the gland after 23 intravenous ascorbate infusions. In some areas of the prostate, SUV was reduced by up to 37% (range 10% to 37%) after treatment. These observations suggested that the rate of cell

membrane synthesis had been decreased by the intravenous ascorbic acid infusions.

Analysis

[^{11}C]acetate-PET/CTAC scans were able to detect the interval change in [^{11}C]acetate uptake by tumor cells before and after 23 intravenous

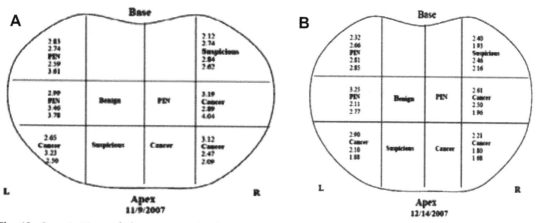

Fig. 12. Case 4. Maps of the prostate gland postoperative pathologic grading with overlay of [^{11}C]acetate metabolic activity in SUVs before (*A*) and after (*B*) ascorbate therapy showing positive correlation with cell atypia and SUV elevation of [^{11}C]acetate before ascorbate therapy and interval reduction in SUV after ascorbate therapy.

ascorbate infusions. Based on the dramatic reduction in tumor metabolism resulting from ascorbate treatment observed in the patient, the authors recommend translating into clinical trials the knowledge gained from the compelling basic science research and case reports in the literature regarding the use of this treatment, perhaps using functional molecular imaging as a measure of response to these novel therapies.

SUMMARY

This article has attempted to provide a brief overview of the relevant imaging modalities available to clinicians to aid in diagnosing, staging, and assessing therapeutic response in prostate cancer (see **Fig. 1**). Advanced imaging techniques allow clinicians to precisely target potential biopsy sites and to objectively assess the course of disease and response to therapy. These imaging techniques have wide-ranging utility, whether using TRUS to guide biopsies or to assess recurrence in the prostate bed; using MRI to assess the location of prostate cancer within the gland itself for biopsy or preoperative planning; or using bone scans, CT scans, and [^{11}C]acetate-PET/CTAC to evaluate for the occurrence of regional or distant metastases. Rather than just observing elevated serum PSA values yet being blind to the potential manifestations that an elevated value may represent in a given patient, these advanced imaging techniques provide clinicians with targeted tools to use in diagnosing, treating, and managing prostate cancer, the number one cancer and number two cancer killer of men.

ACKNOWLEDGMENTS

Acknowledgment to the following staff members of the Division of Nuclear Medicine of the Department of Radiology and the Nuclear Pharmacy Division of the Department of Pharmacy at Kansas University Medical Center: Christine McMillin, RT, CNMT; James Traylor, CNMT; Mark Murphy, MS; John Ternus, RPh; Randy Osburn; and David McKee. A medical writing consultant, Dr Linda A. Landon of Research Communiqué, LLC, provided copyediting of the authors' original text, literature database management, and computer graphic arts production of figures and tables using the authors' original data.

REFERENCES

1. American Cancer Society. Cancer facts and figures 2010. Atlanta (GA): American Cancer Society; 2010.

2. National Institutes of Health. Estimates of funding for various research, condition, and disease categories (RCDC). Bethesda (MD): U.S. Department of Health & Human Services; 2011.

3. Andriole GL, Grubb RL, Buys SS, et al. Mortality results from a randomized prostate-cancer screening trial. N Engl J Med 2009;360(13):1310–9.

4. Schröder FH, Hugosson J, Roobol MJ, et al. Screening and prostate-cancer mortality in a randomized european study. N Engl J Med 2009;360(13):1320–8.

5. Schaffer D, Pendergrass H. Comparison of enzyme, clinical, radiographic, and radionuclide methods of detecting bone metastases from carcinoma of the prostate. Radiology 1976;121(2):431–4.

6. Miller P, Eardley I, Kirby R. Prostate specific antigen and bone scan correlation in the staging and monitoring of patients with prostatic cancer. Br J Urol 1992;70(3):295–8.

7. Rudoni M, Antonini G, Favro M, et al. The clinical value of prostate-specific antigen and bone scintigraphy in the staging of patients with newly diagnosed, pathologically proven prostate cancer. Eur J Nucl Med 1995;22(3):207–11.

8. Gleave M, Coupland D, Drachenberg D, et al. Ability of serum prostate-specific antigen levels to predict normal bone scans in patients with newly diagnosed prostate cancer. Urology 1996;47(5):708–12.

9. Rydh A, Tomic R, Tavelin B, et al. Predictive value of prostate-specific antigen, tumour stage and tumour grade for the outcome of bone scintigraphy in patients with newly diagnosed prostate cancer. Scand J Urol Nephrol 1999;33(2):89–93.

10. Chybowski F, Keller J, Bergstralh E, et al. Predicting radionuclide bone scan findings in patients with newly diagnosed, untreated prostate cancer: prostate specific antigen is superior to all other clinical parameters. J Urol 1991;145(2):313–8.

11. Sabbatini P, Larson S, Kremer A, et al. Prognostic significance of extent of disease in bone in patients with androgen-independent prostate cancer. J Clin Oncol 1999;17(3):948–57.

12. Schirrmeister H, Guhlmann A, Elsner K, et al. Sensitivity in detecting osseous lesions depends on anatomic localization: planar bone scintigraphy versus 18F PET. J Nucl Med 1999;40(10):1623–9.

13. Even-Sapir E, Metser U, Mishani E, et al. The detection of bone metastases in patients with high-risk prostate cancer: 99mTc-MDP Planar bone scintigraphy, single- and multi-field-of-view SPECT, 18F-fluoride PET, and 18F-fluoride PET/CT. J Nucl Med 2006;47(2):287–97.

14. Rinnab L, Blumstein NM, Mottaghy FM, et al. 11C-Choline positron-emission tomography/computed tomography and transrectal ultrasonography for staging localized prostate cancer. BJU Int 2007; 99(6):1421–6.

15. Scattoni V, Montorsi F, Picchio M, et al. Diagnosis of local recurrence after radical prostatectomy. BJU Int Mar 2004;93(5):680–8.

16. Testa C, Schiavina R, Lodi R, et al. Prostate cancer: sextant localization with MR imaging, MR spectroscopy, and 11C-choline PET/CT1. Radiology 2007; 244(3):797–806.

17. Beheshti M, Imamovic L, Broinger G, et al. 18F choline PET/CT in the preoperative staging of prostate cancer in patients with Intermediate or high risk of extracapsular disease: a prospective study of 130 patients. Radiology 2010;254(3):925–33.

18. Pieterman RM, Putten JW, Meuzelaar JJ, et al. Preoperative staging of non–small-cell lung cancer with positron-emission tomography. N Engl J Med 2000;343(4):254–61.

19. Watanabe H, Kanematsu M, Kondo H, et al. Preoperative detection of prostate cancer: a comparison with 11C-choline PET, 18F-fluorodeoxyglucose PET and MR imaging. J Magn Reson Imaging 2010;31(5):1151–6.

20. Albrecht S, Buchegger F, Soloviev D, et al. (11)C-acetate PET in the early evaluation of prostate cancer recurrence. Eur J Nucl Med Mol Imaging 2007;34(2):185–96.

21. Heesakkers RAM, Hövels AM, Jager GJ, et al. MRI with a lymph-node-specific contrast agent as an alternative to CT scan and lymph-node dissection in patients with prostate cancer: a prospective multicohort study. Lancet Oncol 2008;9(9):850–6.

22. Ponsky L, Cherullo E, Starkey R, et al. Evaluation of preoperative ProstaScint scans in the prediction of nodal disease. Prostate Cancer Prostatic Dis 2002; 5(2):132–5.

23. Soloviev D, Fini A, Chierichetti F, et al. PET imaging with 11C-acetate in prostate cancer: a biochemical, radiochemical and clinical perspective. Eur J Nucl Med Mol Imaging 2008;35(5):942–9.

24. Oyama N, Akino H, Kanamaru H, et al. 11C-acetate PET imaging of prostate cancer. J Nucl Med 2002; 43(2):181–6.

25. Haseman MK. Capromab pendetide imaging of occult lymph node metastases. J Nucl Med 1998;39(4):653.

26. Oyama N, Miller TR, Dehdashti F, et al. 11C-acetate PET imaging of prostate cancer: detection of recurrent disease at PSA relapse. J Nucl Med 2003;44(4): 549–55.

27. Stephenson AJ, Kattan MW, Eastham JA, et al. Defining biochemical recurrence of prostate cancer after radical prostatectomy: a proposal for a standardized definition. J Clin Oncol 2006;24(24): 3973–8.

28. Roach M, Hanks G, Thames H, et al. Defining biochemical failure following radiotherapy with or without hormonal therapy in men with clinically localized prostate cancer: recommendations of the RTOG-ASTRO phoenix consensus conference. Int J Radiat Oncol Biol Phys 2006;65(4):965–74.

29. Chen Q, Espey MG, Sun AY, et al. Ascorbate in pharmacologic concentrations selectively generates ascorbate radical and hydrogen peroxide in extracellular fluid in vivo. Proc Natl Acad Sci U S A 2007;104(21):8749–54.

30. Chen Q, Espey MG, Sun AY, et al. Pharmacologic doses of ascorbate act as a prooxidant and decrease growth of aggressive tumor xenografts in mice. Proc Natl Acad Sci U S A 2008;105(32): 11105–9.

31. Hoffer LJ, Levine M, Assouline S, et al. Phase I clinical trial of i.v. ascorbic acid in advanced malignancy. Ann Oncol 2008;19(11):1969–74.

32. Padayatty SJ, Sun AY, Chen Q, et al. Intravenous use by complementary and alternative medicine practitioners and adverse effects. PLoS One 2010; 5(7):e11414.

33. Levine M, Padayatty SJ, Espey MG. Vitamin C: a concentration-function approach yields pharmacology and therapeutic discoveries. Adv Nutr 2011; 2:78–88.

34. Leung K. [11C] Acetate. [Internet]. Vol Created: December 8, 2005; Last Update: May 19. In: National Center for Biotechnology Information, editor. Molecular imaging and contrast agent database (MICAD). Bethesda (MD): National Library of Medicine (US); 2008. p. 2004–9.

Heart Health = Urologic Health and Heart Unhealthy = Urologic Unhealthy: Rapid Review of Lifestyle Changes and Dietary Supplements

Mark A. Moyad, MD, MPH[a,b,]*

KEYWORDS

• Heart • Urology • Lifestyle change • Dietary supplements

Almost all aspects of urology are affected by lifestyle changes and dietary supplements.[1–3] Yet, putting a quick summary together of these interventions is a daunting task because some of these interventions have potential profound impacts independently or in combination with conventional therapy, others have no impact, and some could negatively affect treatment and overall health. Over the last decade, few specialties have arguably invested more energy and effort in determining whether or not certain dietary supplements affect a variety of medical conditions than urology.[4,5] Thus, a quick review of potentially efficacious and nonefficacious lifestyle and supplemental interventions seems necessary.

BENIGN PROSTATIC HYPERPLASIA

Benign prostatic hyperplasia (BPH) or lower urinary tract symptoms have a long history of being positively affected by heart-healthy lifestyle changes. Thus, reminding patients that almost anything heart healthy is prostate healthy is a simplistic and important mantra.[6] Conversely, heart-unhealthy changes increase the risk of exacerbation of BPH, such as

lack of exercise, obesity, excess alcohol intake, poor mental health, high cholesterol level, heart disease, hypertension, diabetes, tobacco use, and so forth, which all seem to have a potential profound impact via multiple mechanisms, including increased sympathetic tone, cholesterol, oxidative stress, and so forth.[7–15]

β-Sitosterol and Other Cholesterol Reducers

Phytosterols are found in a variety of plants and plant oils.[16] Phytosterols are similar in structure to cholesterol except for a minor structural difference. Phytosterols are not synthesized in humans and are not well absorbed, are excreted more rapidly from the liver than cholesterol, and are not found in high concentrations in human tissues. The main phytosterols found in the diet are sitosterol, stigmasterol, and campesterol. β-Sitosterol is the phytosterol found in largest quantity in the diet. Phytosterols block the uptake of exogenous cholesterol from dietary and bile sources in the intestinal tract. Low-density lipoprotein (LDL) cholesterol is reduced by phytosterols, and high-density lipoprotein (HDL) and triglycerides are not affected. The blockage of cholesterol absorption may produce a relative

a Department of Urology, University of Michigan Medical Center, 1500 East Medical Center Drive, Ann Arbor, MI 48109-0330, USA
b Eisenhower Wellness Institute, Eisenhower Medical Center, Rancho Mirage, CA, USA
* Department of Urology, University of Michigan Medical Center, 1500 East Medical Center Drive, Ann Arbor, MI 48109-0330.
E-mail address: moyad@umich.edu

Urol Clin N Am 38 (2011) 359–367
doi:10.1016/j.ucl.2011.05.004

cholesterol pool reduction, which is followed by upregulation of cholesterol synthesis and LDL receptors, which can increase LDL removal. This process is similar to how some healthy dietary fats found in many healthy foods, such as almonds or pistachios, may also reduce LDL levels and improve some specific urologic outcomes.[17,18]

More than 40 clinical trials of phytosterols have been conducted that have ranged from 1 to 12 months.[16,19,20] Plant sterols added to foods such as yogurt, margarine, orange juice, mayonnaise, milk, and olive oil have been shown to reduce LDL level by approximately 10% to 15% (mean of 10%–11%) when approximately 2000 mg/d is ingested. About 1600 to 3000 mg of plant sterol supplemental or tablet consumption can also reduce LDL levels by approximately 4% to 15%. Plant sterols may also reduce the absorption of some fat-soluble vitamins; so, there has been some debate as to whether multivitamins should be consumed with the use of these products.

The primary mode of action of these sterols via cholesterol uptake reduction and a minor antiinflammatory mechanism suggests, in my opinion, that they are weaker mimics of the drug ezetimibe (Zetia), which can reduce LDL levels by approximately 20% with a 10-mg dose.[21,22] Recently, laboratory research has demonstrated the ability of ezetimibe to favorably affect prostate tissue and reduce BPH.[23] Ezetimibe is commonly added to statin therapy or other lipid-lowering agents to achieve synergistic impacts and, more favorably, reduce LDL level.[21,22] Therefore, it should not be surprising that β-sitosterol by itself or with other cholesterol-lowering medications could favorably affect BPH. For example, despite some data that suggest no impact of statins on established BPH over a short period,[24,25] other new epidemiologic and past laboratory studies suggest potentially favorable impacts on BPH prevention and progression with cholesterol-lowering prescribed medications.[26–28]

Two meta-analyses, performed by similar investigators in 1999 and 2000, suggested that β-sitosterol could provide some benefit for men with BPH.[29,30] In some of these studies, β-sitosterol is an extract that contains a variety of phytosterols or plant cholesterols that are usually derived from the South African star grass (Hypoxis rooperi). Researchers reported an impressive mean difference compared with placebo; the International Prostate Symptom Score was −4.9 points, peak urinary flow rate was 3.91 mL/s, and residual volume was −28.62 mL. β-Sitosterol did not affect prostate size, which is of interest because there is some preliminary evidence that it may mildly inhibit 5α-reductase.[31] The withdrawal rates were similar to those of placebo (approximately 8%). Most common side effects

with β-sitosterol were gastrointestinal side effects in 1.6% and erectile dysfunction in 0.5%. These analyses were conducted from 4 trials that involved 519 men. The question is to why not try β-sitosterol, a heart health ingredient, with or without medications for BPH. The dosage range in these studies has been from 0.30 mg of β-sitosterol-β-D-glucoside to approximately 200 mg/d. However, the dosage recommended in cholesterol treatment guidelines is 2000 to 3000 mg a day to reduce LDL by 6% to 15%, and, in fact, these National Cholesterol Education Panel recommendations state that "Plant stanol/sterol esters (2 g/day) are a therapeutic option to enhance LDL cholesterol lowering."[32] However, no recent studies of β-sitosterol have been published, but, if a patient is going to use a cost-effective product for cholesterol reduction, it is theoretically possible that a secondary benefit may be prevention or reduction in some aspect of BPH.

A 2002 meta-analysis of 18 Pygeum africanum clinical trials suggested a potential benefit with this supplement.[33] These compounds are an extract of the African prune tree. The mean duration of clinical studies was 64 days, but men were more than 2 times as likely to report an improvement in overall symptoms; nocturia was reduced by 19%, residual volume was reduced by 24%, and peak urine flow was increased by 23%. The withdrawal rate was similar to placebo at 12%. Adverse effects were similar to those of placebo, and the most frequently reported adverse effects were gastrointestinal. Most studies used a standardized extract effective at approximately 100 to 200 mg/d. One of the main components of Pygeum africanum and saw palmetto are phytosterols that include β-sitosterol.[34,35] However, the problem with Pygeum is demand compared with precious supply, in that the bark is derived from an endangered tree.[36] This is not the case with saw palmetto, which seems to be in abundance and has arguably a diverse number of heart-healthy compounds beyond β-sitosterol, including the primary monounsaturated fat found in olive oil (oleic acid) and a variety of other potentially healthy dietary fats that may have the ability to increase HDL levels and lower cardiovascular events.[37–40]

CHRONIC NONBACTERIAL PROSTATITIS AND INTERSTITIAL CYSTITIS

Dietary supplements in chronic nonbacterial prostatitis and interstitial cystitis are actually fairly well known and have a history of being heart healthy, and some even reduce blood pressure in prehypertensive patients.[41–45] Less known is that there is a history of some heart-healthy lifestyle changes that have also displayed some preliminary profound effects.

A randomized double-blinded lifestyle clinical study from Florence, Italy, had impressive results because the participants were previously unresponsive to conventional treatments.[46] Participants (average age of 36–38 years, body mass index [BMI, calculated as the weight in kilograms divided by height in meters squared] of 22, mean symptom duration of 5.5–6 months) had symptoms of pain in the pelvic region for 3 or more months continuously and scored a minimum of 15 points on the National Institutes of Health–Chronic Prostatitis Symptom Index (NIH-CPSI) with at least 6 or more points on the pain subscale. A total of 52 subjects were placed in the exercise group and 51 were assigned to the placebo/stretching group. The outcome measures were the NIH-CPSI, the Beck Depression Inventory, the State Anxiety Inventory-Y, and a pain visual analog scale (VAS). These evaluations were determined at baseline and 6 and 18 weeks. The exercise group engaged in vigorous walking 3 times per week for 40 minutes of each session to achieve 70% to 80% of the predicted maximum heart rate for their age. The placebo/stretching group did a series of stretching exercises but had to maintain their heart rate below 110 beats per minute for the entire session. Approximately 25% of the participants dropped out of the study by 18 weeks. However, significant differences between the 2 groups favored the exercise group for total NIH-CPSI ($P = .006$), pain ($P = .0009$), quality-of-life subscales ($P = .02$), and VAS ($P = .003$). No difference was found for other parameters. Responders were considered those who experienced a decrease of 6 or more points in total NIH-CPSI (58% exercise vs 43% placebo), 25% to 49% (39% vs 35%), and a decrease of 50% (19% vs 5%) or more from baseline in total NIH-CPSI. A placebo response of 25% of this magnitude is expected from other trials. Pain is the symptom that is the most influential variable and the quality-of-life predictor and should be one of the main targets of any therapy. Exercise induces release of endogenous opioids and reduces sympathetic activity to the prostate.[47–49]

KIDNEY/BLADDER/PROSTATE CANCERS

One of the strongest correlations for any cancer risk or progression and smoking is not just lung cancer but bladder cancer.[50,51] In addition, smoking after bladder or prostate cancer treatment may also increase the risk of cancer recurrence and heart disease.[50–52] Obesity is linked to multiple cancers, but kidney cancer (renal cell) has arguably the strongest correlation of almost any cancer type in terms of a higher risk with

a greater BMI or waist circumference.[53–56] Hypertension, lack of exercise, smoking, and even dyslipidemia may also be associated with increased risks of kidney cancer. Almost every heart-healthy behavior that one can imagine is associated with a potential lower risk of prostate cancer.[1,2] Few medical specialties seem to have such a close correlation with cardiovascular health and risk compared with urology.

In terms of dietary supplementation, there is evidence to suggest that high doses of or megadosing on most dietary supplements or antioxidants does not seem to provide benefit and may even encourage tumor growth in some cases.[4,57–69] This evidence is similar to the evidence that has already existed in terms of cardiovascular risk increases with larger intakes of dietary supplements.[63–65]

In a small and randomized study from the 1990s, there was a suggestion that megadoses of a supplement as opposed to a recommended daily allowance (RDA) supplement may reduce the risk of non–muscle-invasive bladder cancer recurrence after BCG treatment.[70] However, a larger follow-up study was needed to confirm these preliminary findings, which recently occurred.[71] Patients who were BCG naive with carcinoma in situ, Ta bladder cancer, or T1 bladder cancer were randomized to receive intravesical BCG or BCG plus interferon alfa-2b and then further randomized to receive an RDA (minimal intake) or megadose supplement. Each RDA tablet of vitamins contained 25% of the recommended daily dose, and patients took 2 tablets twice daily of either the RDA or the megadose supplement. Each megadose tablet contained 9000 IU of vitamin A, 25 mg of vitamin B6, 500 mg of vitamin C, 400 IU of vitamin D3, 400 μg of folate, 100 IU of vitamin E, and 7.6 mg of zinc. Induction BCG was given weekly for 6 weeks and then at 4, 7, 13, 19, 25, and 37 months. The primary end point was biopsy-confirmed recurrence or cytology that was positive. A total of 670 patients were randomized, and, at a 24-month median follow-up, there were no significant differences between the RDA and megadose supplements groups. The following recurrence-free survival numbers were BCG + RDA, 63%; BCG + megadose supplement, 59%; BCG + interferon + RDA, 55%; and BCG + interferon + megadose supplement, 61%. Megadose supplements and/or interferon alfa-2b added to BCG did not affect time to recurrence in patients with non–muscle-invasive bladder cancer. Also, there was a slight nonsignificant increased risk of recurrence with BCG and the megadose supplement.

When the first study was published in the 1990s in the *Journal of Urology*, it was visionary,[70] and megadose vitamins probably did reduce the risk of recurrence in my opinion. Why? Researchers were arguably dealing with a population of individuals that had deficiencies in a variety of vitamins and minerals. Fast-forward almost 2 decades later and patients are not deficient but seem to be over-supplemented with antioxidants from foods, beverages, and supplements.[72] This oversupplementation makes it difficult to truly conduct a large clinical trial of a truly deficient healthy population over a long period, despite some investigators calling for the need for such studies[73] because when these clinical trials are designed, deficiencies are more prevalent, but, by the time the trial commences, the deficiencies may no longer exist. In addition, in the more recent bladder cancer trial, the megadose supplement itself had added folic acid and vitamin D to it compared with the original formulation used in the preliminary successful study.[70,71] Why was the formula altered from what was potentially successful in the preliminary study because of some minimal laboratory and population data? Would this formula be allowed in definitive phase 3 pharmaceutical studies in which the phase 1 or 2 had a successful outcome and safety with a specific dose and formulation, which was altered in the phase 3 trial? Arguably these nutrients, especially folic acid, also have data to suggest that they could also increase recurrence of certain cancers or other abnormalities when given at these higher doses.[4,57–69] Lower doses of these supplements may be providing the benefits needed without adding the significant increased risks or overall concerns for most individuals.[74,75] Over the past 20 years, multiple randomized trials and some observational studies suggest that a potentially heart- and digestive-healthy probiotic found in some types of yogurt and available as potential dietary supplement may reduce the risk of bladder cancer or recurrence after conventional treatment.[76–81]

INFERTILITY AND SEXUAL DYSFUNCTION

Heart-unhealthy behaviors also negatively affect male fertility.[82] Obesity, high cholesterol and blood pressure, lack of exercise, improper diet, stress, depression, and multiple other cardiovascular risk factors that increase oxidative stress all have some minor or major impact on fertility and are arguably the most holistic approach to changing patients lives and improving overall outcomes.[83,84] Authoritative medical reviews have suggested that antioxidant supplement treatment could be considered a primary treatment of some male

fertility issues.[85] In addition, a recent Cochrane review is one of the most extensive published data on male fertility and dietary supplements because it reviewed 34 clinical trials with 2876 couples.[86] The overall findings concluded that antioxidant supplementation in men seems to have a positive role in improving the outcomes of live birth and pregnancy rates in couples participating in assisted reproduction techniques. The *P* values for live births and pregnancy rates were .0008 and .00001, respectively. Critics of this analysis on live births also arguably point toward the small number of such events (n = 20) that occurred from a total of 214 couples in only 3 studies that was used in this part of the analysis or the pregnancy rates that actually were derived from 96 pregnancies in 15 trials that included 964 couples. Yet, it is still relevant that this is a viable minimal or moderate option for some men, given the low cost of most antioxidants used in these studies. In addition, adverse events were similar to those of a placebo, with no serious adverse events reported in any trial.

Which specific dietary supplements and at what dosage and frequency should be recommended for male fertility issues? This extensive Cochrane review could not identify one superior individual antioxidant or combination product from these trials,[86] so clinicians and patients are left with questions. In my opinion, the supplements that have a past overall safety record that may be heart healthy should be the only ones recommended for fertility from this past review,[86] especially if there is equivalent efficacy among all the trials with positive results, in other words, coenzyme Q10 at 200 to 300 mg/day,[87] L-carnitine at 2000 to 3000 mg/d,[88–92] ω-3 fatty acids (fish oil),[93–95] and vitamin C[96–98] but not high-dose supplements that have a potential heart-unhealthy or overall male-unhealthy profile such as folic acid,[57–60] selenium, and vitamin E,[4,61–63] or even megadoses of zinc.[67]

One of the more overt examples of heart-healthy lifestyle changes positively affecting urologic health has to be in male and female sexual dysfunction.[99–103] These changes can also improve the efficacy of prescription erectile dysfunction medications.[104] This category is one of the easiest for the reader to locate healthy lifestyle and supplement recommendations in the medical literature, which shows how far this area of urology has progressed.

SUMMARY

Heart healthy seems tantamount to overall urologic health. This concept also potentially seems to be the case for kidney stones or choosing a supplement that could be used with conventional treatment of Peyronie disease.[105–109] It seems that large and diverse (the American Cancer Society, the American Heart Association, and the American Diabetes Association) health care preventive organizations are beginning to apply this same concept[110] because neither the truly life-changing lifestyle recommendations nor the dietary supplements for patients are mutually exclusive in my opinion. These lifestyle changes and dietary supplements affect a variety of potential clinical end points and have the highest overall probability of affecting all-cause mortality. This effect is critical in my opinion because again the forest has to take precedence over the tree to improve the overall state of urologic health. The less a clinician wants to focus on these issues, the less I also believe that patients will respond to them, and, even worse, the more likely in my opinion, patients will begin to listen to less-credible sources for guidance.[111] This latter choice is simply not acceptable; however, this abnormal situation has become so common today in other nonurologic areas that it is almost considered normal for some patients to take lifestyle, supplement, and general preventive advices from the person at the counter of the local health food store over their practitioner. Perhaps this article is a simple small step in the appropriate direction. Heart health = urologic health should be the unified mantra for urologic practitioners because it is easy to construe for patients, is simple and fast for the clinician to recommend, and arguably has the best chance of immediately improving the lives of patients.

REFERENCES

1. Moyad MA. Step-by-step lifestyle changes that can improve urologic health in men, part I: what do I tell my patients? Prim Care 2006;33:139–63.
2. Moyad MA. Step-by-step lifestyle changes that can improve urologic health in men, part II: what do I tell my patients? Prim Care 2006;33:165–85.
3. Moyad MA. Calcium oxalate kidney stones: another reason to encourage moderate calcium intakes and other dietary changes. Urol Nurs 2003;23:310–3.
4. Lippman SM, Klein EA, Goodman PJ, et al. Effect of selenium and vitamin E on risk of prostate cancer and other cancers: the Selenium and Vitamin E Cancer Prevention Trial (SELECT). JAMA 2009;301:39–51.
5. Lee J, Andriole G, Avins A, et al. Redesigning a large-scale clinical trial in response to negative external trial results: the CAMUS study of phytotherapy for benign prostatic hyperplasia. Clin Trials 2009;6:628–36.
6. Moyad MA. Lifestyle changes to prevent BPH: heart healthy = prostate healthy. Urol Nurs 2003; 23:439–41.
7. Parsons JK. Lifestyle factors, benign prostatic hyperplasia, and lower urinary tract symptoms. Curr Opin Urol 2011;21:1–4.
8. Moyad MA, Lowe FC. Educating patients about lifestyle modifications for prostate health. Am J Med 2008;121(8 Suppl 2):S34–42.
9. Sea J, Poon KS, McVary KT. Review of exercise and the risk of benign prostatic hyperplasia. Phys Sportsmed 2009;37:75–83.
10. Mongiu AK, McVary KT. Lower urinary tract symptoms, benign prostatic hyperplasia, and obesity. Curr Urol Rep 2009;10:247–53.
11. Wong SY, Woo J, Leung JC, et al. Depressive symptoms and lifestyle factors as risk factors of lower urinary tract symptoms in Southern Chinese men: a prospective study. Aging Male 2010;13:113–9.
12. Zhang X, Zhang J, Chen J, et al. Prevalence and risk factors of nocturia and nocturia-related quality of life in the Chinese population. Urol Int 2011;86: 173–8.
13. Parsons JK, Im R. Alcohol consumption is associated with a decreased risk of benign prostatic hyperplasia. J Urol 2009;182:1463–8.
14. Parsons JK, Bergstrom J, Barrett-Connor E. Lipids, lipoproteins and the risk of benign prostatic hyperplasia in community-dwelling men. BJU Int 2008; 101:313–8.
15. Parsons JK. Modifiable risk factors for benign prostatic hyperplasia and lower urinary tract symptoms: new approaches to old problems. J Urol 2007;178: 395–401.
16. Jones PJ, AbuMweis SS. Phytosterols as functional food ingredients: linkages to cardiovascular disease and cancer. Curr Opin Clin Nutr Metab Care 2009; 12:147–51.
17. Berryman CE, Preston AG, Karmally W, et al. Effects of almond consumption on the reduction of LDL-cholesterol: a discussion of potential mechanisms and future research directions. Nutr Rev 2011;69:171–85.
18. Aldemir M, Okulu E, Neselioglu S, et al. Pistachio diet improves erectile function parameters and serum lipid profiles in patients with erectile dysfunction. Int J Impot Res 2011;23:32–8.
19. Guardamagna O, Abello F, Baracco V, et al. Primary hyperlipidemias in children: effect of plant sterol supplementation on plasma lipids and markers of cholesterol synthesis and absorption. Acta Diabetol 2011;48:127–33.
20. Malinkowski JM, Gehret MM. Phytosterols for dyslipidemia. Am J Health Syst Pharm 2010;67:1165–73.
21. Hamilton P. Role of ezetimibe in the management of patients with atherosclerosis. Coron Artery Dis 2009;20:169–74.

22. Dujovne CA, Suresh R, McCrary Sisk C, et al. Safety and efficacy of ezetimibe monotherapy in 1624 primary hypercholesterolaemic patients for up to 2 years. Int J Clin Pract 2008;62:1332–6.

23. Pelton K, Di Vizio D, Insabato L, et al. Ezetimibe reduces enlarged prostate in an animal model of benign prostatic hyperplasia. J Urol 2010;184:1555–9.

24. Mills IW, Crossland A, Patel A, et al. Atorvastatin treatment for men with lower urinary tract symptoms and benign prostatic enlargement. Eur Urol 2007;52:503–9.

25. Stamatiou KN, Zaglavira P, Skolarikos A, et al. The effects of lovastatin on conventional medical treatment of lower urinary tract symptoms with finasteride. Int Braz J Urol 2008;34:555–61.

26. Hall SA, Chiu GR, Link CL, et al. Are statin medications associated with lower urinary tract symptoms in men and women? Results from the Boston Area Community Health (BACH) Survey. Ann Epidemiol 2011;21:149–55.

27. St Sauver JL, Jacobsen SJ, Jacobson DJ, et al. Statin use and decreased risk of benign prostatic enlargement and lower urinary tract symptoms. BJU Int 2011;107:443–50.

28. Padayatty SJ, Marcelli M, Shao TC, et al. Lovastatin-induced apoptosis in prostate stromal cells. J Clin Endocrinol Metab 1997;82:1434–9.

29. Wilt TJ, MacDonald R, Ishani A. Beta-sitosterol for the treatment of benign prostatic hyperplasia: a systematic review. BJU Int 1999;83:976–83.

30. Wilt T, Ishani A, MacDonald R, et al. Beta-sitosterols for benign prostatic hyperplasia. Cochrane Database Syst Rev 2000;2:CD001043.

31. Cabeza M, Bratoeff E, Heuze I, et al. Effect of beta-sitosterol as inhibitor of 5-alpha-reductase in hamster prostate. Proc West Pharmacol Soc 2003;46:153–5.

32. National Cholesterol Education Porgram (NCEP) Expert Panel on Detection, Evaluation, and Treatment of High Blood Cholesterol in Adults (Adult Treatment Panel III). Third report of the National Cholesterol Education Program (NCEP) Expert Panel on Detection, Evaluation, and Treatment of High Blood Cholesterol in Adults (Adult Treatment Panel III) final report. Circulation 2002;106:3143–421.

33. Wilt T, Ishani A, Mac Donald R, et al. *Pygeum africanum* for benign prostatic hyperplasia. Cochrane Database Syst Rev 2002;1:CD001044.

34. McQueen CE, Bryant PJ. Pygeum. Am J Health Syst Pharm 2001;58:120–3.

35. Suzuki M, Ito Y, Fujino T, et al. Pharmacological effects of saw palmetto extract in the lower urinary tract. Acta Pharmacol Sin 2009;30:227–81.

36. Stewart KM. The African cherry (*Prunus africana*): can lessons be learned from an over-exploited tree. J Ethnopharmacol 2003;89:3–13.

37. Lopez-Miranda J, Perez-Jimenez F, Ros E, et al. Olive oil and health: summary of the II international conference on olive oil and health consensus report, Jaen and Cordoba (Spain) 2008. Nutr Metab Cardiovasc Dis 2010;20:284–94.

38. Mensink RP, Zock PL, Kester AD, et al. Effects of dietary fatty acids and carbohydrates on the ratio of serum total to HDL cholesterol and on serum lipids and apolipoproteins: a meta-analysis of 60 controlled trials. Am J Clin Nutr 2003;77:1146–55.

39. Kochikuzhyil BM, Devi K, Fattepur SR. Effect of saturated fatty acid-rich dietary vegetable oils on lipid profile, antioxidant enzymes and glucose tolerance in diabetic rats. Indian J Pharmacol 2010;42:142–5.

40. Yamagishi K, Iso H, Yatsuya H, et al, JACC Study Group. Dietary intake of saturated fatty acids and mortality from cardiovascular disease in Japanese: the Japan Collaborative Cohort Study for Evaluation of Cancer Risk. Am J Clin Nutr 2010;92:759–65.

41. Shoskes DA, Zeitlin SI, Shahed A, et al. Quercetin in men with category III chronic prostatitis: a preliminary prospective, double-blind, placebo-controlled trial. Urology 1999;54:960–3.

42. Wagenlehner FM, Schneider H, Ludwig M, et al. A pollen extract (Cernilton) in patients with inflammatory chronic prostatitis-chronic pelvic pain syndrome: a multicentre, randomized, prospective, double-blind, placebo-controlled phase 3 study. Eur Urol 2009;56:544–51.

43. Asakawa K, Nandachi N, Satoh S, et al. Effects of cernitin pollen extract (Cernilton) on inflammatory cytokines in sex-hormone-induced nonbacterial prostatitis rats. Hinyokika Kiyo 2001;47:459–65 [in Japanese].

44. Katske F, Shoskes DA, Sender M, et al. Treatment of interstitial cystitis with a quercetin supplement. Tech Urol 2001;7(1):44–6.

45. Boots AW, Haenen GR, Bast A. Health effects of quercetin: from antioxidant to nutraceutical. Eur J Pharmacol 2008;585:325–37.

46. Giubilei G, Mondaini N, Minervini A, et al. Physical activity of men with chronic prostatitis/chronic pelvic pain syndrome not satisfied with conventional treatments—could it represent a valid option? The physical activity and male pelvic pain trial: a double-blind, randomized study. J Urol 2007;177:159–65.

47. Pool JL. Role of sympathetic nervous system in hypertension and benign prostatic hyperplasia. Br J Clin Pract Suppl 1994;74:13–7.

48. McVary KT, Rademaker A, Lloyd GL, et al. Autonomic nervous system overactivity in men with lower urinary tract symptoms secondary to benign prostatic hyperplasia. J Urol 2005;174(4 Pt 1):1327–433.

49. Esch T, Stefano GB. The neurobiology of stress management. Neuro Endocrinol Lett 2010;31:19–39.

50. Grossman HB, Stenzl A, Moyad MA, et al. Bladder cancer: chemoprevention, complementary approaches and budgetary considerations. Scand J Urol Nephrol Suppl 2008;218:213–33.

51. Vilensky D, Lawrentschuk N, Hersey K, et al. A smoking cessation program as a resource for bladder cancer patients. Can Urol Assoc J 2011;1–7. [Epub ahead of print].

52. Joshu CE, Mondul AM, Meinhold CL, et al. Cigarette smoking and prostate cancer recurrence after prostatectomy. J Natl Cancer Inst 2011;103: 835–8.

53. Lipworth L, Tarone RE, McLaughlin JK. Renal cell cancer among African Americans: an epidemiologic review. BMC Cancer 2011;11:133.

54. Chow WH, Dong LM, Devesa SS. Epidemiology and risk factors for kidney cancer. Nat Rev Urol 2010;7:245–57.

55. Moyad MA. Obesity, interrelated mechanisms, and exposures and kidney cancer. Semin Urol Oncol 2001;19:270–9.

56. Khurana V, Caldito G, Ankem M. Statins might reduce risk of renal cell carcinoma in humans: case-control study of 500,000 veterans. Urology 2008;71:118–22.

57. Cole BF, Baron JA, Sandler RS, et al, Polyp Prevention Study Group. Folic acid for the prevention of colorectal adenomas: a randomized clinical trial. JAMA 2007;297:2351–9.

58. Figueriredo JC, Grau MV, Haile RW, et al. Folic acid and risk of prostate cancer: results from a randomized clinical trial. J Natl Cancer Inst 2009;101: 432–5.

59. Collin SM, Metcalfe C, Refsum H, et al. Circulating folate, vitamin B12, homocysteine, vitamin B12 transport proteins, and risk of prostate cancer: a case-control study, systematic review, and meta-analysis. Cancer Epidemiol Biomarkers Prev 2010; 19:1632–42.

60. Bailey RL, Mills JL, Yetley EA, et al. Unmetabolized serum folic acid and its relation to folic acid intake from diet and supplements in a nationally representative sample of adults aged > or=60 y in the United States. Am J Clin Nutr 2010;92:383–9.

61. Duffield-Lillico AJ, Slate EH, Reid ME, et al, Nutritional Prevention of Cancer Study Group. Selenium supplementation and secondary prevention of non-melanoma skin cancer in a randomized trial. J Natl Cancer Inst 2003;95:1477–81.

62. Stranges S, Marshall JR, Natarajan R, et al. Effects of long-term selenium supplementation on the incidence of type 2 diabetes: a randomized trial. Ann Intern Med 2007;147:217–23.

63. Miller ER 3rd, Pastor-Barriuso R, Dalal D, et al. Meta-analysis: high-dosage vitamin E supplementation may increase all-cause mortality. Ann Intern Med 2005;142:37–46.

64. Clarke R, Halsey J, Lewington S, et al, B-vitamin Treatment Trialists' Collaboration. Effects of lowering homocysteine levels with B vitamins on cardiovascular disease, cancer, and cause-specific mortality. Meta-analysis of 8 randomized trials involving 37,485 individuals. Arch Intern Med 2010;170: 1622–31.

65. Sesso HD, Buring JE, Christen WG, et al. Vitamins E and C in the prevention of cardiovascular disease in men: the Physicians' Health Study II randomized controlled trial. JAMA 2008;300:2123–33.

66. Moyad MA. Selenium and vitamin E supplements for prostate cancer: evidence or embellishment? Urology 2002;59(4 Suppl 1):9–19.

67. Moyad MA. Zinc for prostate disease and other conditions: a little evidence, a lot of hype, and a significant potential problem. Urol Nurs 2004; 24:49–52.

68. Giovannucci E, Chan AT. Role of vitamin and mineral supplementation and aspirin use in cancer survivors. J Clin Oncol 2010;28:4081–5.

69. Lawson KA, Wright ME, Subar A, et al. Multivitamin use and risk of prostate cancer in the National Institutes of Health-AARP Diet and Health Study. J Natl Cancer Inst 2007;99:754–64.

70. Lamm DL, Riggs DR, Shriver JS, et al. Megadose vitamins in bladder cancer: a double-blind clinical trial. J Urol 1994;151:21–6.

71. Nepple KG, Lightfoot AJ, Rosevear HM, et al. Bacillus Calmette-Guérin with or without interferon alpha-2b and megadose versus recommended daily allowance vitamins during induction and maintenance intravesical treatment of nonmuscle invasive bladder cancer. J Urol 2010;184:1915–9.

72. Moyad MA. Dr Moyad's no bogus science health advice. Ann Arbor (MI): Ann Arbor Media Group; 2009.

73. Morris MC, Tangney CC. A potential design flaw of randomized trials of vitamin supplements. JAMA 2011;305:1348–9.

74. Tighe P, Ward M, McNulty H, et al. A dose-finding trial of the effect of long-term folic acid intervention: implications for food fortification policy. Am J Clin Nutr 2011;93:11–8.

75. Hercberg S, Galan P, Preziosi P, et al. The SU.VI.MAX study: a randomized, placebo-controlled trial of the health effects of antioxidant vitamins and minerals. Arch Intern Med 2004;164:2335–42.

76. Aso Y, Akazan H. Prophylactic effect of a Lactobacillus preparation on the recurrence of superficial bladder cancer. BLP Study Group. Urol Int 1992; 49:125–9.

77. Aso Y, Akaza H, Kotake T, et al, BLP Study Group. Preventive effect of a Lactobacillus casei preparation on the recurrence of superficial bladder cancer in a double-blind trial. Eur Urol 1995;27:104–9.

78. Naito S, Koga H, Yamaguchi A, et al, Kyushu University Urological Oncology Group. Prevention

of recurrence with epirubicin and lactobacillus casei after transurethral resection of the bladder. J Urol 2008;179:485–90.

79. Ohashi Y, Nakai S, Tsukamoto T, et al. Habitual intake of lactic acid bacteria and risk reduction of bladder cancer. Urol Int 2002;68:273–80.

80. Larsson SC, Andersson SO, Johansson JE, et al. Cultured milk, yogurt, and dairy intake in relation to bladder cancer risk in a prospective study of Swedish women and men. Am J Clin Nutr 2008; 88:1083–7.

81. di Giuseppe R, Di Castelnuovo A, Melegari C, et al, on behalf of the Moli-sani Project Investigators. Typical breakfast food consumption and risk factors for cardiovascular disease in a large sample of Italian adults. Nutr Metab Cardiovasc Dis 2010 Nov 17. [Epub ahead of print].

82. Cabler S, Agarwal A, Flint M, et al. Obesity: modern man's fertility nemesis. Asian J Androl 2010;12: 480–9.

83. Kasturi SS, Tannir J, Brannigan RE. The metabolic syndrome and male infertility. J Androl 2008;29:251–9.

84. Campagne DM. Should fertilization treatment start with reducing stress? Hum Reprod 2006;21:1651–8.

85. Agarwal A, Sekhon LH. The role of antioxidant therapy in the treatment of male infertility. Hum Fertil (Camb) 2010;13:217–25.

86. Showell MG, Brown J, Yazdani A, et al. Antioxidants for male subfertility. Cochrane Database Syst Rev 2011;1:CD007411.

87. Littarru GP, Tiano L. Clinical aspects of coenzyme Q10: an update. Nutrition 2010;26:250–4.

88. Balercia G, Regoli F, Armeni T, et al. Placebo-controlled double-blind randomized trial on the use of L-carnitine, L-acetylcarnitine, or combined L-carnitine and L-acetylcarnitine in men with idiopathic asthenozoospermia. Fertil Steril 2005;84: 662–71.

89. Lenzi A, Lombardo F, Sgro P, et al. Use of carnitine therapy in selected cases of male factor infertility: a double-blind crossover trial. Fertil Steril 2003; 79:292–300.

90. Li Z, Chen GW, Shang XJ, et al. A controlled randomized trial of the use of combined L-carnitine and acetyl-L-carnitine treatment in men with oligoasthenozoospermia. Zhonghua Nan Ke Xue 2005;11:761–4 [in Chinese].

91. Peivandi S, Abasali K, Narges M. Effects of L-carnitine on infertile men's spermogram: a randomized clinical trial. J Reprod Infertil 2010;10:331.

92. Lombardo F, Gandini L, Agarwal A, et al. A prospective double blind placebo controlled cross over trial of carnitine therapy in selected cases of male infertility. Fertil Steril 2002;78(Suppl 1):68–9.

93. Marchioli R, Barzi F, Bomba E, et al. Early protection against sudden cardiac death by n-3 polyunsaturated fatty acids after myocardial infarction: time-course analysis of the results of the Gruppo Italiano per lo Studio della Sopravvivenza nell'Infarto Miocardico (GISSI)-Prevenzione. Circulation 2002;105:1897–903.

94. Matsuzaki M, Yokoyama M, Saito Y, et al, JELIS investigators. Incremental effects of eicosapentaenoic acid on cardiovascular events in statin-treated patients with coronary artery disease. Circ J 2009; 73:1283–90.

95. Conquer JA, Martin JB, Tummon I, et al. Effect of DHA supplementation on DHA status and sperm motility in asthenozoospermic males. Lipids 2000; 35:149–54.

96. Colagar AH, Marzony ET. Ascorbic acid in human seminal plasma: determination and its relationship to sperm quality. J Clin Biochem Nutr 2009;45: 144–9.

97. 6 Vitamin C content in foods. Available at: http://www.vitamincfoundation.org/usda.html. Accessed March 20, 2011.

98. Moyad MA, Combs MA, Baisley JE, et al. Vitamin C with metabolites: additional analysis suggests favorable changes in oxalate. Urol Nurs 2009;29: 383–5.

99. Esposito K, Giugliano F, Di Palo C, et al. Effect of lifestyle changes on erectile dysfunction in obese men. JAMA 2004;291(24):2978–84.

100. Giugliano D, Giugliano F, Esposito K. Sexual dysfunction and the Mediterranean diet. Public Health Nutr 2006;9:1118–20.

101. Hannan JL, Maio MT, Komolova M, et al. Beneficial impact of exercise and obesity interventions on erectile function and its risk factors. J Sex Med 2009;6(Suppl 3):254–61.

102. Horasanli K, Boylu U, Kendirci M, et al. Do lifestyle changes work for improving erectile function? Asian J Androl 2008;10:28–35.

103. Esposito K, Maiorino MI, Bellastella G, et al. Determinants of female sexual dysfunction in type 2 diabetes. Int J Impot Res 2010;22:179–84.

104. Maio G, Saraeb S, Marchiori A. Physical activity and PDE5 inhibitors in the treatment of erectile dysfunction: results of a randomized controlled study. J Sex Med 2010;7:2201–8.

105. Reiner AP, Kahn A, Eisner BH, et al. Kidney stones and subclinical atherosclerosis in young adults: the CARDIA Study. J Urol 2011;185:920–5.

106. Siener R, Jansen B, Watzer B, et al. Effect of n-3 fatty acid supplementation on urinary risk factors for calcium oxalate stone formation. J Urol 2011; 185:719–24.

107. Taylor EN, Stampfer MJ, Mount DB, et al. DASH-style diet and 24-hour urine composition. Clin J Am Soc Nephrol 2010;5:2315–22.

108. Taylor EN, Fung TT, Curhan GC. DASH-style diet associates with reduced risk for kidney stones. J Am Soc Nephrol 2009;20:2253–9.

109. Safarinejad MR. Safety and efficacy of coenzyme Q10 supplementation in early chronic Peyronie's disease: a double-blind, placebo-controlled randomized study. Int J Impot Res 2010;22:298–309.

110. Eyre H, Kahn R, Robertson RM, et al, ACS/ADA/AHA Collaborative Writing Committee Members. Preventing cancer, cardiovascular disease, and diabetes: a common agenda for the American Cancer Society, the American Diabetes Association, and the American Heart Association. Circulation 2004;109:3244–55.

111. Mills E, Ernst E, Singh R, et al. Health food store recommendations: implications for breast cancer patients. Breast Cancer Res 2003;5(6):170–4.

Index

Note: Page numbers of article titles are in **boldface** type.

urologic.theclinics.com

Printed and bound by CPI Group (UK) Ltd, Croydon, CR0 4YY

03/10/2024

01040360-0002